ENOUGH IS ENOUGH

How the Soveya Solution is Revolutionizing the Diet and Weight-Loss World

ELI GLASER, CNWC, CWMS

FOREWORD BY *Dr. David Lieberman,*
N Y TIMES BESTSELLING AUTHOR

outskirts press

Enough is Enough
How the Soveya Solution is Revolutionizing the Diet and Weight-Loss World

v4.0

Outskirts Press, Inc.
http://www.outskirtspress.com

Paperback ISBN: 978-1-4787-6488-5
Hardback ISBN: 978-1-9772-1349-5

Library of Congress Control Number: 2019907503

PRINTED IN THE UNITED STATES OF AMERICA

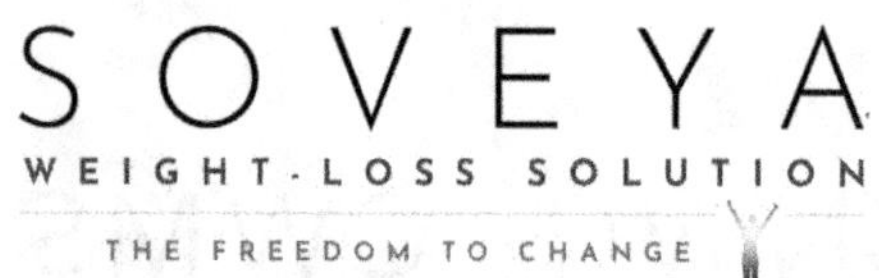

695 Cross Street, Suite 190
Lakewood, NJ 08701
1.888.8.SOVEYA (876.8392)
www.soveya.com
info@soveya.com

NOTE FROM THE AUTHOR

This book is not intended to provide medical advice, a diagnosis or treatment for any condition. It is offered for educational and informative purposes only. Always seek the guidance of a qualified health-care provider before making any changes to your diet, or with any questions regarding a medical condition or treatment. Do not disregard medical advice or delay seeking it or avoid or delay treatment because of something you read in this book. You are encouraged to share the information in this book with your health-care provider and to access any resource necessary to improve your nutrition, health and wellness.

SOVEYA SUCCESS STORIES

"When they found a carcinoid tumor on my appendix, it motivated me to do something significant about my health. I wanted to put healthier food in my body (especially because of the correlation between cancer and sugar intake). I turned to Soveya at the recommendation of a friend. I trusted Eli because he has sustained a 100-pound weight loss for years, was a certified nutritionist, and brings a different perspective. I knew losing weight wasn't just a matter of learning which foods were the right ones to eat; I needed something deeper. I wanted real, sustained change. I needed a coach, like anyone who wants to achieve any results that are currently beyond his or her grasp.

On our first call, I shared with him about my life as a mom of two young boys, a wife, and a volunteer executive director of a non-profit. I had a long list of valid reasons for why I made the choices I made with my time and energy. Eli listened kindly and then shared with me the following idea. Some people define wisdom as knowing the difference between what is important and what is not important. But the real definition of wisdom is knowing the difference between what's important and what's more important. Everything I am doing is important. But caring for myself is actually more important.

I began weeping. I could suddenly see how much was really depending on me taking care of myself. I could see how much it was hurting me when I behaved like I am disposable and not worth the effort. I could see how I was failing my children when I gave up on myself. Through continued coaching with Eli, ranging from the emotional to the practical, I lost more than twenty-five pounds and have kept it off for seven years. I am grateful that I am continuing to use the food plan and am maintaining a healthy weight. I truly love the Soveya plan because it is flexible enough to allow me to eat every type of food (sans flour and sugar) but gives me boundaries that I need to stay healthy forever."

- Erica, Washington, D.C.

"At age 29, I weighed 350 pounds. My eating was out of control. My clothes did not fit and I was out of breath after walking up just 5 stairs. I had tried many diets in the past – none had any permanent results. In fact, the weight came back faster than I was able to lose it. I did not want to talk to anyone about my weight problem. On the outside, I was a successful teacher, with a great wife and family. On the inside, I was ashamed and lonely.

Then I met Eli. He was the first person that I had spoken to who actually understood what I was going through, because he went thru it himself. He understood my problem. He told me he lost a lot of weight and was keeping it off. I thought he was lying, but then he went on to explain that the solution is more than changing what and how you eat. I was not quite sure what he meant, but I listened to him and followed what he told me to do because I was desperate for help.

The result: I lost 150 pounds and have kept it off for 10 years now. Eli is easy to talk to, has great suggestions and is a soothing, comforting voice that has helped me achieve this goal. Not only have I had physical results, but I also have seen improvement in my relationship with my wife, children and colleagues at work. I attribute all this to the advice and suggestions that Eli has given me.

Eli understands the pain of someone who can't stop eating. The solution he offers works. I am living proof. If I can do it, anyone can."

- Barry, Passaic, New Jersey

"I would like to express my profound gratitude to you. So much goodness has resulted in my life, and my husband's, because of Soveya. Between the two of us, we have lost well over one hundred pounds and kept it off for eleven years. Calm and confidence are now in my being, and these go deeper than ever before. My thoughts are not wrapped up in food. How can I ever thank you enough for this? I thank you for the freedom I feel. In the past, holidays were an excuse to eat until I was stuffed. I really hated myself afterwards. But I couldn't stop the cycle. How grateful I am to Soveya for helping me stop that cycle."

- Paula, Jerusalem, Israel

"You were really amazing at explaining everything to me and my daughter. When I came home, I told my husband that you were worth every penny! The whole afternoon, we were reviewing what we learned today. She even insisted on making a salad from the cookbook which we all enjoyed for dinner!

I have always been wary of setting too many limits on food for my daughter, because I was worried of negative emotional effects. I was very reassured by the warmth and positivity with which you presented the information to her. She is very enthusiastic to go on this journey which is such a relief for me! Thank you."

- Chaya, Baltimore, Maryland

TABLE OF CONTENTS

FOREWORD

DR. DAVID LIEBERMAN

Eli gets it.

Eli understands the failure and frustration of dieting because he was a frequent flyer on the weight-loss rollercoaster for many years, losing and gaining so often that he earned himself what seemed like a lifetime pass. But it certainly wasn't free. In fact, it nearly cost him his health.

At a morbidly obese 300 pounds, his struggles with overeating were significant but not uncommon. His physical and emotional discomfort were profound and personal, but not unusual. Two out of every three people in this country are either overweight or obese. Those who don't fight the battle of the bulge are the exception, not the norm.

That's one reason why he is such an effective weight-loss coach. He can intimately relate to his clients and they can relate to him. He has first-hand experience with the overwhelming cravings and temptations, the temporary hope and the devastating despair. He lived the life that so many people still do and made the lifestyle changes that so many desperately desire—but so few have.

Eli gets the fact that long-term weight loss is not about crash dieting or merely counting calories. He recognizes the real issues and fundamental problems people need to address, because he went through it himself—and has been residing at the same location of a healthy body size for the past seventeen years. He has no plans to move anytime soon.

And Eli has the honesty, courage and credibility to confront the billion-dollar weight-loss industry. He is exposing the misleading messaging, defying the distorted mindset and challenging the broken methodology that is so rampant in so much of conventional dieting. His message and method is clear, concise, and current: that we have to once-and-for-all stop focusing on just changing our weight and start focusing on changing ourselves and our relationship with food. To finally acknowledge that the only quick fix is to admit that there is no quick fix.

But Eli also gives it.

In addition to his personal experience and clinical accreditation, Eli possesses a unique and transformative three-dimensional skill set. He is a seasoned and skilled educator, an enlightening and engaging communicator and an effective and empowering coach. As he likes to call himself: the CCO–Chief Change Officer.

His dynamic and compelling style is complemented by his completely down-to-earth and relatable personality, allowing him to deal with this sensitive subject in a disarming and non-judgmental manner. Eli simultaneously creates an atmosphere of comfort and commitment whether working one-to-one or in a room with hundreds.

Eli has developed a proven and practical system that has impacted thousands of people around the world. The Soveya Solution pinpoints the vital areas upon which a person has to focus in order to effect real and lasting success. It's a constructive and comprehensive approach to weight loss, providing concrete tools, guidelines, and procedures applicable for anyone willing to step outside of their comfort zone, learn new behaviors, and challenge their previously held beliefs about dieting.

I can professionally and personally attest to the impact and efficacy of Eli's approach. I've seen his work first hand and have witnessed how people have changed their attitudes toward food and relationship with eating and self-indulgence. It's a learning and growth process that is not always easy but forever rewarding. Now, with the publication of this book, Eli's message and methodology will be available to millions more. And it's also a really good read.

I highly recommend the Soveya Solution to anyone who is looking for a long-term answer to what has been a lifelong problem. It's the first and last book you'll need to buy about diet and weight loss. Because the Soveya Solution is not just a weight-changer, and it's not even a game- changer. It's a life-changer.

David J. Lieberman. Ph.D. is an award-winning author and internationally recognized leader in the fields of human behavior and interpersonal relationships. Techniques based on his 11 books, which have been translated into 27 languages and include two New York Times bestsellers, are used by the FBI, The Department of the Navy, Fortune 500 companies, and by governments and corporations in more than 25 countries. He has appeared as a guest expert on more than 300 programs such as The Today Show, Fox News, and The View, and his work has been featured in publications around the world. Dr. Lieberman, whose Ph.D. is in psychology, lectures and holds workshops across the country on a variety of topics.

drdavidlieberman.com

ACKNOWLEDGEMENTS

A cook creates the meal, and the waiter serves it. I consider myself a waiter much more than a cook.

I don't take credit for originating all of the underlying principles and ideas offered in these pages. I've had the incredible pleasure and privilege of having been exposed to so many wise and wonderful "chefs" from so many different walks of life. Their boundless knowledge, insight, and personal experiences have nourished and enriched me beyond description. Real soul food.

I'm eternally grateful that I had the wisdom and willingness to be receptive to the teachings and life lessons they were so generous and gracious to share. That, I'll take credit for.

I also take my job as a waiter very seriously. I'm committed to serving these truths in the most engaging, impactful and transformative way possible. No paper plates or plastic cutlery here. My singular goal is for anyone who reads this book—no matter your background or body size—to be more nourished and knowledgeable as a result. Just like putting down the fork after the last bite of a delicious and nutritious meal leaves you energized, satisfied, and gratified, so too is my wish for you upon turning over the last page.

These past seventeen years have been a true growth experience – in addition to losing 130 pounds and being smart enough to not try and find them. I can't help but look back on the long and winding road that has brought me to this point and acknowledge the people that have empowered me along the way.

I changed careers after changing my life – earned my nutrition certification and provide weight-loss coaching and inspirational seminars to thousands of people all over the world. Whether in front of one person or a hundred, my message is always the same: successful weight loss is not about losing weight; it's about changing your relationship with food – and yourself.

That's the theme I want to share with you between the covers of this book – so you can go under your covers tonight feeling better about yourself, tucked in with the tenets to begin your own journey toward healthy eating, to fall asleep on a pillow filled firmly with practical tools, clear direction, and achievable goals – not stuffed with hot air and empty promises.

I'm forever indebted to Kevin, a diehard Pats fan who

promised me nothing more than the experience, strength, and hope he embodied and that I could replicate if I had the humility to accept his sound and straightforward suggestions. I'm so glad I had the clarity to clear the cotton out of my ears and absorb his advice. I guess you could say it was a clean handoff, and I've been running with the ball ever since.

Speaking of running, I'd be remiss if I didn't reveal my respect and appreciation to my running coach, Chana B. who, with her husband Neil have—without exaggeration--volunteered years of their time to helping others reach abstinence, serenity, and success.

My first exposure to highly successful businessmen, particularly Arnie Polinger, Rick Zitelman, and Dennis Berman taught me that "doing good and being good" is not a just a theoretical concept. They are exceptional men who are exceptionally generous with their time, resources, and expertise. They knew me "when" and could see through the 130 pounds of my added exterior into my inner potential.

Abe Fenster, David Dannenbaum, and Mort Fertel were three ad-hoc mentors who – through the sheer kindness of their hearts and sweetness of their souls—added so many seeds of sagacity over so many hours of their valuable time, wanting nothing in return other than to see the Soveya Solution to take root and blossom. I'm so appreciative of their green thumbs and request forgiveness for not formulating the fortitude to cultivate their plantings sooner.

The same sentiments go out to all of my clients who nudged, insinuated, and insisted that I put pen to paper in order to create a medium for the Soveya message and method to be shared with so many more. "Eli, you've gotta write this book. It will change the world," was a refrain I received often from my very supportive chorus. Working with all of you has greatly helped me polish and fine tune the notes on the following sheets, which I hope is melodious and moving music to everyone's ears. Special shout out to Lorry L., who edited my first very rough scores.

The galvanizing kick in the pants was proffered from my personal and professional relationship with Sandy Feder, whose business coaching and consulting skills are highly credible, concrete, and convincing. He did for me what I do for others, namely corralling my courage to conquer my comfort zone and step into the brave new world of risk and reward.

I've had the rewarding experience of associating with accomplished and talented business associates, Dr. David Lieberman being one of them. I am very appreciative that he agreed to author the foreword to this book.

I've had the unbelievable blessing of benefiting from the wisdom, guidance, and counsel of a multitude of teachers, but especially from Rabbi Noach Orlowek, whose otherworldly ability to simultaneously be a father, brother, leader, and sage is eclipsed only by the unconditional love and compassion with which he tenders his caring touch.

I've been fortunate to be friended by the finest of fellows, none more open-handed and open-hearted than my bosom buddy, Michael Stern, who tragically passed away shortly before the publication of this book. All the merit garnered as a result of anyone benefiting from this work should be credited toward the honor and elevation of his blessed memory. That list of comrades in arms is also topped by my two "partners in crime," Ira Trocki and Sender Rochwarger, who – with their wonderful wives—have shared their most prized possessions, their son and daughter as spouses for my kids.

My children, son-in-law, daughter-in-law, and grandkids are sources of unlimited pleasure and purpose in my life. I pray that I adequately fulfill my role as your father and properly appreciate the amazing gifts and joy you provide to your parents and to mankind. We are all so much better off for having all of you in the world.

One might say that the most useless tool in the world is a compass. What's it created to do? Point to the North Pole. But of the millions of people who have ever purchased this contraption, how many of them were heading to the North Pole? Zero. Exactly. So, what's the point?

The answer is that even though that's what it's built to do, that's not really its construct. The purpose of a compass is to show direction, not necessarily to identify a location. That, in fact, is an incredibly important function in life, because we all need direction and guidance on our wonderful and unique journeys.

My wife, Zakah, is the compass for our family – as well as for countless others around the world. Her caring, courage, consistency, and commitment have blazed personal and professional paths of success and achievement that myriads of people pine to imitate. She magnificently manages her roles as wife, mother, sister, daughter, executive, mentor and friend – making us all feel loved and valued while still insisting we turn off the light in the kitchen before going to bed. She is my role model for personal growth and is the foundation upon with the Soveya Solution rests.

All of these gifts have been undeservedly bestowed upon me by my Father in Heaven, to Whom I am forever beholden. I strive to utilize the skills and abilities vested in me to continually improve myself and help perfect the world – one pound at a time.

This book is dedicated to my dear parents.

My mother-in-law, Dorothy Hinde, whose unconditional support, love and generosity flows uninterrupted from the ever-open valve in her huge heart. May she continue to experience good health and great joy from her family for many years to come.

To my father and mother, of blessed memory, who gave me so much in such different ways. The drive to learn, teach and explore, to better myself by helping others emanated from their genuine and selfless desire to make a distinct and decisive difference in this world. I hope that my efforts afford them eternal satisfaction and pride.

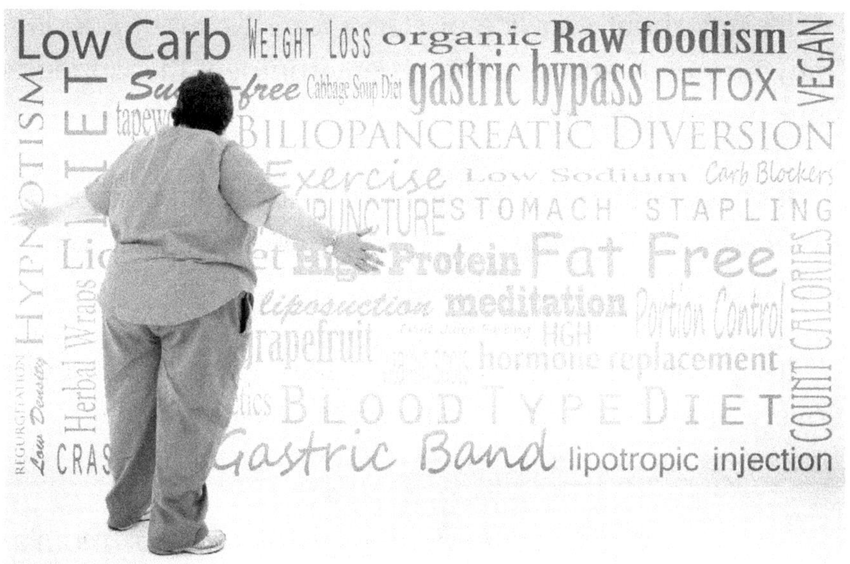

1

THE SOVEYA SOLUTION

Successful weight loss is not about *losing weight*. It's about developing a *healthy relationship with food*.

It's not about *ketosis, calculating calories*, or *counting points*. It's about *honesty, consistency,* and *accountability*.

It's not about *willpower*. It's about a *willingness* to learn new behaviors, embrace change and be teachable at whatever age and stage of life you're in.

It's not about *sacrifice* or *starvation*. It's about *prioritizing your needs* and creating an environment that supports your new way of life.

It's not about being *strong* or *strict*. It's about being *comfortable* and *committed* to eat appropriately when others aren't, or refrain while others indulge.

It's not about the newest fad, biggest loser, or latest discovery of a miracle fat-burning plant. It's about turning the *burden* to say "no" into the *freedom* to say "no."

It's not just about *information, inspiration,* or *motivation*. It's about TRANSFORMATION.

It's about the courage to conquer your fears and step outside your comfort zone.

Get off the dieting rollercoaster, already. ***Enough is finally enough.***

If you really want to once and for all meet your goals – to not just lose weight but *maintain* a healthy body size—then you must stop focusing on changing your *weight* and start focusing on changing *yourself.*

That's where the **Soveya Solution** comes in.

It's a clear, concise and comprehensive system that helps you confront that "four-letter" word that intimidates us all: C-H-A-N-G-E.

THE SOVEYA SYSTEM FOR SUCCESS:

ONE FOUNDATION – THREE PILLARS – SEVEN KEYS

It starts with the *foundation*—to develop and sustain a healthy relationship with food.

A Healthy relationship with food is built on three *pillars*: Your Head, your Heart, and your Hands. Those are the three target areas of change. Without addressing all three, it's just a recipe for relapse and formula for failure.

Your head is your attitude and understanding – having an intellectual clarity as to the purpose of eating and function that food is meant to fulfill. Changing your whole mindset about dieting is crucial as well as overhauling the language of weight loss. It's not about being perfect. It's about being precise. It's not about failure. It's about being focused and seeing that your daily relationship with food is the essential element in your overall health and wellness.

Your heart is having a healthy and mature emotional association with food. To break free from the overwhelming feeling of dependency on the immediate gratification, comfort, escape, or indulgence eating plays in your life.

Your hands are your actions – what foods you should eat, how much and when. A well-defined food plan with clear goals, guidelines, and boundaries that is customized exclusively for you – and that can adapt to your changing schedule, situation, and station in life.

So far, so good. Sounds simple and straightforward. Not so fast. Why? Because so many of us have one or more blocks that are preventing us from making these necessary changes.

And that's where the seven Soveya keys come in – to help you unlock your blocks and to pinpoint your personal impediments. To push yourself past your comfort zone and embrace the freedom to change.

Changing your eating habits and relationship with food can seem overwhelming – it's not a piece of cake to not take that piece of cake. It's much easier and more comfortable to act on instinct and feed your immediate gratifications.

Adhering to boundaries – whether that means holding yourself back or pushing yourself forward—requires intellectual, emotional, and physical effort that your mind and body often don't want to exert. Change is challenging. Inertia is inviting.

But you have a choice: to either endure the discomfort of discipline or the comfort of complacency, which in the end isn't so comfortable at all. You have a choice to break out of your own personal comfort zone to meet and maintain your genuine goals or continue feeding on the bitter dessert of regret and remorse.

A RELATIONSHIP WITH *FOOD*?

Aren't relationships between people, who exchange ideas, feelings, and have mutual interests? What do I possibly have in common with spaghetti squash?

It turns out, one of the most intimate and indispensable relationships every human being has is with food. Eating is the most important thing we do every day to keep ourselves alive. None of us can opt out and not be adversely affected. Nobody can take a pass and expect not to eventually pass out. It's one of the most fundamental rules of nature: A human being must eat to live – but not live to eat.

And therefore, developing and maintaining a healthy relationship with food is critical for all of us. No one is exempt.

A healthy relationship with food is to see food for what it is, and what it isn't. A healthy relationship with food is to have healthy boundaries around eating; to neither overeat nor under eat. Enough really is enough.

A healthy relationship with food is to invest in and prioritize self-love and self-care through proper nutrition, not self-indulgence, self-medication, or self-sacrifice.

We are otherwise intelligent and accomplished people. We're good folks. Yet, why do we do this to ourselves? Why is it so darn hard? Because food, especially unhealthy food, can be an intense, palatable pleasure. It's a fun, enjoyable, mouthwatering experience. We're not eating to live, we're living to eat – more aptly, literally dying for that next bite.

So, is the solution to make eating a robotic, perfunctory daily occurrence, void of any pleasure? Absolutely not. The answer is to prioritize between function and fun; not that function has to rule out fun, but it has to rule over fun.

The function of our eating should be to give us health and wellbeing. This is the primary purpose of food – a delivery system for nutrients that provide our bodies the energy, health and vitality to live. That mindset should direct our choices. That's the bedrock for a healthy relationship with food, one that also gives us the greatest pleasure, both in the short term and long term.

Let's finally get off the runaway roller coaster that is career dieting, continually going up and down the scale, gaining and losing weight so often that our closets are filled with clothes that span the many sizes our girth has grown and shrunk, akin to a second-hand department store for which we are the only unsatisfied customer. Come on, already, enough is enough!

Weight loss is a multi-billion-dollar industry--not because we're given hidden wisdom, before which was accessible only to a select few, but rather because the majority of us are incapable of sticking with a diet program for any extended length of time because we're not given the tools to institute a significant life change with our behavior with food.

That's why a comprehensive approach addressing our attitude and emotions around food – in addition to our actions--is critical. Successful weight loss can be achieved only in the context of an overall makeover of our relationship with eating, to satisfy and invigorate our physical needs instead of indulging our immediate gratifications or medicating and suppressing our emotional distress.

Let's face it. We've all got issues. Whether it's parents, children, spouses, bosses, or friends; money, prestige, career, school, or simply getting out of the front door each day; every one of us has things that can cause stress and anxiety. Some more, some less.

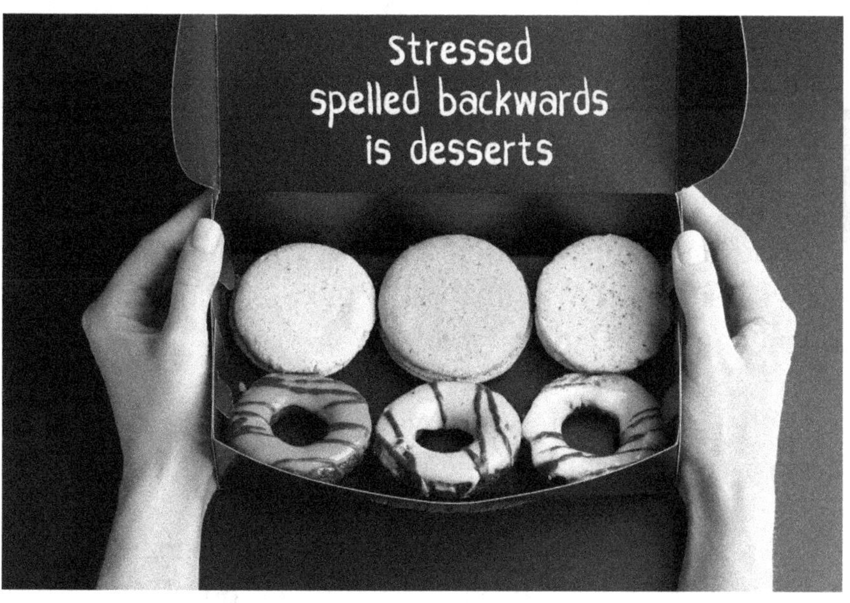

And many of us turn to food. It's an easy emotional elixir. Fritos instead of feelings.

It's as close as my refrigerator or corner store. There's a lot of it. It's legal. From the TV ads to the billboards, it's constantly being shoved in our collective face. Who can't recite by heart a jingle for some famous food or drink? It's literally ingrained in our national psyche. And it tastes good. Sooo good.

It's not the perfect recipe; it's the perfect storm.

The mega diet business is counter balanced only by the super-sized food advertising and marketing world. Those of us simultaneously struggling with weight and temptation are caught in this cataclysmic catch-22; a bruised and battered ping-pong ball being paddled back and forth by industry giants milking us for our last dollar and ounce of sanity. A suspicious cynic would conclude they're working in cahoots to insure a healthy supply of unhealthy customers.

And the solutions offered mostly miss the main point. Why? Because they primarily focus on salving the consequence, not solving the problem.

What I'm about to share with you now may seem quite controversial. But I'm going to do it anyway. Ready?

Obesity is not a *medical* problem – it's a *behavior* problem. It's not a *weight* problem, it's a *food* problem.

How can I say that when being overweight is among the leading causes of heart disease, high blood pressure, high cholesterol, stroke, diabetes, and several forms of cancer – not to mention scores of chronic ailments and conditions? Aren't we literally killing ourselves with our forks and knives?

Absolutely. But the answer is that these deadly risks directly associated with weight gain and obesity are a result of our eating behaviors and lifestyle choices. They are the consequences of our actions. And if we want to take them seriously and effort to eradicate them, then we must focus on solving the problem.

Please don't misunderstand me. I'm not discouraging anyone from going to a doctor. It's essential to seek medical help for any kind of illness. It's the responsible and prudent thing to do. Some of my best friends and family members are highly competent and caring health-care professionals. But even a bariatric surgeon will tell you that the long-term efficacy of any invasive weight-loss procedure is dependent on the patient changing their eating behaviors and relationship with food.

Now this all may sound like a theoretical game of semantics. But it's not. It's the fundamental difference between success and failure when it comes to losing weight.

The primary reason that the weight-loss recidivism rate is so high (some claim it to be more than 90%) is because we're investing our time, energy, hopes, and money in dealing with the consequences, instead of focusing on solving the problem. It's like an alcoholic downing a pot of black coffee, getting sober, and proclaiming that he's cured and that it will never happen again. He temporarily took care of his inebriation, but he didn't address the underlying problem. So, what will inevitably occur? He'll get drunk again.

It's like putting a Band-Aid on a sore and thinking that will cure the infection. Going on a diet is like going in a cold shower after night of boozing – it could sober you up – or take off the pounds – but won't stop you from running back to the bar – or to the buffet.

The only formula for long-term success is to identify the core problem and apply a remedy to that issue.

So, what's our problem? We have an unhealthy, dysfunctional relationship with food. That's what we have to focus on. That's what we have to change. And the benefit of developing – and maintaining – a healthy relationship with food is not just losing weight, but keeping it off.

Now, we can become discouraged and depressed by realizing this is a self-inflicted wound or energized and encouraged by understanding that the cure is no further than in our very own head, heart, and hands. We may need a doctor to address the consequences, but it's up to us to solve the problem. There's no surgery or supplement that can alter our attitude or emotions. It's a temptation, not a tumor.

The number one question I'm continually asked is, *"Eli, how have you kept off more than 100 pounds for 17 years? What's your secret?"*

And my answer is always the same: I'm not any stronger or smarter than anyone. It's not about any great self-control. It's all about two words: honesty and maturity. My willingness to engage in unconditional (and sometimes uncomfortable) honesty when it came to my eating habits, and desire to "grow up" and mature in my relationship with self- indulgence and immediate gratification.

Those two characteristics are part and parcel of every human being. Without exception. We all have the ability to be honest with ourselves and to engage in self-maturation. For some of us, it requires more internal digging to uncover those traits. But they are there for all of us to access – and they're worth every single shovelful.

Distinguishing between the problem and the consequence, between the solution and the benefit. This is the formula for long-term success. This is what the Soveya Solution is all about: staying laser focused on the core issue and providing practical and effective tools to solve the problem. And this is why we're creating a revolution in the way the world looks at weight loss.

We're taking the solution out of the grasp of the medical world, advertisers, and supplement suppliers and putting it back where it belongs, in the palm of your hand. Grab hold and don't let go. It'll be an awesome ride.

"These are life-changing tools."

– Brocha, Melbourne, Australia

2

ELI'S STORY: ENOUGH IS ENOUGH

I burst through the front door and headed straight for the fridge with such an intense desire that nothing could get in my way. I was simultaneously drawn relentlessly by food and immobilized to do anything else. I was locked in and zoned out. Little else mattered.

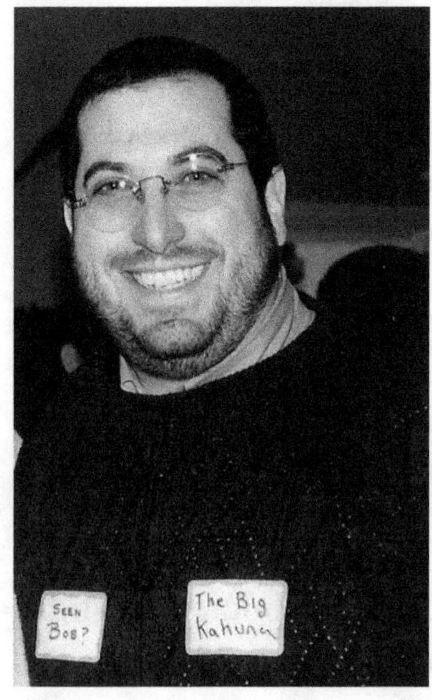

I barely tolerated distractions. I didn't bother to hang my coat in the closet or to look in on the sleeping kids. I dreaded my turn to drive the babysitter home because that meant a five, maybe ten-minute delay from doing what I HAD to do. I HAD to eat!

My wife and I came home Saturday evening from our "date night" out – the one time during the week we could steal away for a few hours. I always enjoyed our time together but was often preoccupied with what was coming: my late-night binge. I was fixated on the leftovers in the fridge: the meatloaf, spaghetti, or homemade apple pie. I was consumed by thoughts of consuming – the ultimate consumer.

Did I feel hungry? Hardly. I had dinner before we left. Did I feel compelled to eat? Absolutely!

Enough was never enough. I couldn't say "no."

Opening the refrigerator door, the subtle sound of the air-tight rubber seal releasing its grip washed over me a fond familiarity – like a comforting sigh of relief you feel taking the first step into your house after returning from a long trip. But for me, the fridge was home.

Out came the food, one container after another. Not sure exactly what I craved, I put it all on the counter, making sure I covered all my bases. I popped off the tops, grabbed a serving bowl from the cabinet and a fork from the drawer. No mere dinner plate was capable of accommodating what I needed.

Brimming full, I put the bowl into the microwave and pressed the buttons. This was one of my biggest dilemmas of the night: should I time it for three minutes to make sure it was plenty hot, or 90 seconds because I couldn't wait. Guess which choice I usually made.

The countdown began. I rushed to get the bottle of *diet* soda, positioning it near the salt, spices, and newspaper, carefully arranging my "shrine to the binge."

70 seconds.

Wherever I was in the kitchen, whatever I was doing, I always had one eye on the clock. Sometimes I just stood and stared at the numbers, captivated by thoughts of getting at my food. 57, 56, 55 . . . .

That wasn't, however, the only thing going on in my mind. For in fact a fierce war was waging between my ears. *Why am I doing this? I'm not hungry. It's midnight. I should just go to bed. I don't need to eat anymore. This is insane.*

I'd even think to myself in the second person. *You know you're going to feel horrible about yourself. You know you're going to be physically uncomfortable, if not sick. You know you're not going to sleep well.*

You're pitiful and lack all self-control.

40, 39, 38, 37 . . . .

The debate sometimes spilled out of my mouth. I'd actually talk out loud as I was preparing the food. "You know that this is not in your best interest," I'd say matter-of-factly, shaking my head while shaking the jar of mayonnaise for the last little gobs. "I don't need to be doing this. Dump out the food. Put it back in the fridge and go to sleep. Enough is enough, already. Just say 'no.'"

I couldn't. I HAD to eat.

15, 14, 13, 12 . . . .

As the time approached my eyes got big, my mouth watering with excitement. I counted down the last ticks of the clock. But guess what — I couldn't even wait for the final bell to ring and yanked open the door.

With the grace and coordination of a seasoned waiter, I pivoted the bowl from the microwave to the table, settling it in the sweet spot of my "shrine." Pulled up the chair, sat down and . . . poof. It was gone.

The bowl was empty, chewing seemed optional. I didn't really enjoy it because I didn't really remember eating it. Inhaling is more accurate. It usually took me less time to consume it than it did to heat it up – although it was rarely more than warm. No sooner did I dive in for the first bite than I stuffed in the last.

And no sooner did I put down the fork from that final bite then the waves of humiliation and disgust overcame me as a just and bitter dessert.

I did it again. That was so ridiculous.

I was humiliated in front of no one but myself. My reality was stark and sad. I was overcome by a piece of flesh from a dead animal and fried vegetable taken from the dirt.

Why can't I control myself? Why can't I just say "no"?

The answer (even though I didn't know it at the time) was painful but simple. I was a compulsive overeater. I was utterly overwhelmed by my desire to indulge with food.

I was a slave to sugar, paralyzed by pizza, and hypnotized by hamburgers. Lots of them. I could eat a whole bucket of fried chicken, or a Pu-Pu platter serving four and still have room for the main course. I craved quantities. I never bothered super-sizing, because I always ordered in plural; two of this and three of that.

Did it bother me that my extreme eating habits elevated my weight to a morbidly obese 300 pounds? For sure. Did it stop me? No.

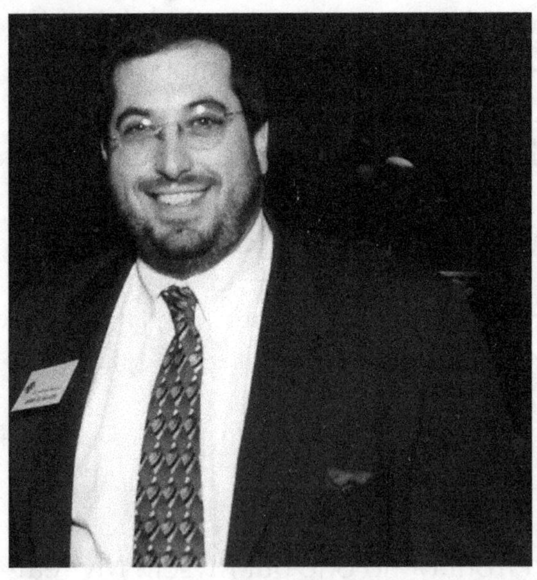

I knew what I was doing. I fancy myself a reasonably intelligent guy. I knew that eating massive quantities of food made me fat, lethargic, physically and emotionally sick. I knew if I ate fruits, vegetables, lean protein, and grains – in reasonable portions – I'd lose weight and gain back my health. But knowing and changing are two very different things. The distance between my head and heart seemed like eighteen miles instead of eighteen inches. When it came to food, "no" was not in my vocabulary.

For years, I ate against my will.

Late-night eating was my favorite. Waking up bloated, gaseous and fatigued from a restless night sleeping on a distended stomach was my norm.

I rarely desired breakfast. Besides, those kinds of foods weren't my cup of tea. But already by 10 o'clock the obsession with lunch started kicking in. No matter what I was doing, or with whom I was talking, food was my focus.

Where was I going to go? What was I going to order? I barely ever brought lunch with me to work. Where was the excitement? Besides, it was limited to the confines of the brown paper bag.

Eating out meant varied and multiple choices. I could satisfy my craving because I could get whatever I wanted and however much I wanted. I ordered from the dinner menu during the day because the lunch specials weren't big enough.

All-you-can-eat buffets were my home away from home; the barbeque grill my most cherished appliance. I would go through three propane canisters in one summer, and we didn't even entertain that often. But when we did, I was in heaven.

Being the grill guy gave me license to binge in broad daylight without anyone seeing – at least that's what I led myself to believe. A cooler packed with meats at my side, I worked the tongs like a master chef, grilling different cuts to people's perfection, and at the same time always having an extra on the fire for myself. I was the hit of the party. Everyone loved their burgers, dogs, or chicken, and I loved pleasing everyone. And, I made sure I was surreptitiously eating along with them, thinking I could blend into the background behind the barbeque.

Then, when the party was slowing down, when everyone else had finished eating, I'd walk out from behind my dugout with a plate full of stuff and sit down to have my "meal."

"Wow, Eli, you're just now going to eat?!" they'd say in admiration, implying that I pushed off my own meal until everyone else got what they needed. I smirked a half-way-acknowledging grin, quickly burying my inner shame with a double burger--fixings spilling over the bun while

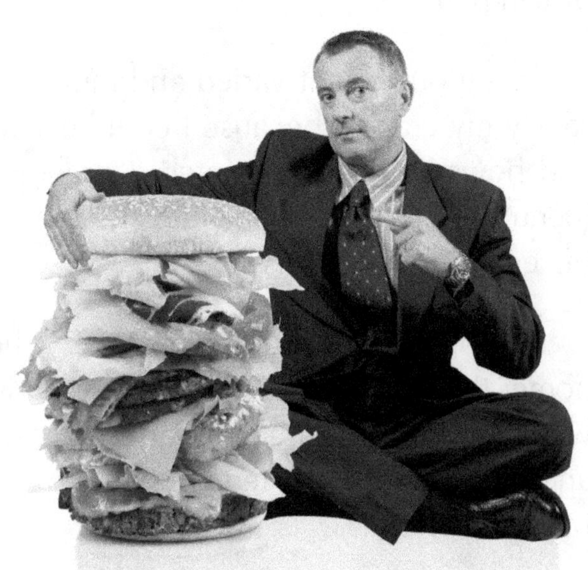

potato salad spilled over the edge of the plate. I would end the day having pounded down pounds and pounds of meat.

Therein lay one of my primary problems: I couldn't differentiate between five ounces and five pounds. I was truly quantitatively challenged. Enough was never, ever enough.

When it came to food, I didn't have a stop sign. The switch in my mind that signaled "enough" didn't work. I valued the meal more by how much I ate than by how much I enjoyed the taste.

Left to my own devices, I would eat until I ran out of time or ran out of money. I'd eat when I was glad, mad, or sad. I'd use food to reward myself and to distract me from things I didn't want to think about – the perfect anesthetic. Fritos instead of feelings.

I would stuff down my emotions with food. I'd medicate with meatballs to avoid dealing with life's issues, secure in the knowledge that I could always write my own prescription. I copped to the cupcakes and caved in to the cravings. I felt entitled to indulge.

I was isolating when it came to meals. I'd purposely come home late for dinner so as not to have to eat with everyone else. I felt a sense of comfort and security eating alone, whether at 8 o'clock at night or 2 o'clock in the morning. At restaurants, I'd always try to find the corner table facing the wall, secluded by a newspaper and my irrational belief that no one would see food for two being served to a table with a place setting for one.

Was I always that way? Yes and no. I grew up riding the diet yoyo, either losing or gaining 10 - 20 pounds. I don't remember ever being able to maintain a consistent weight. Twice in my life, however, I did put on a lot--my first year after high school and my first year after college. Clearly, I didn't do transitions well. I didn't know it at the time. All I knew is that I was 50 pounds overweight and feeling miserable about myself.

I was, however, eventually able to take the weight off on my own. I loved playing sports and was able to use that as motivation to eat normal-sized portions and make good food choices: grilled chicken instead of deep fried; orange slices in place of banana splits, etc. . . . I would play basketball (or whatever sport was in season), or work out in a gym before or after having dinner. I called it "stringing it together." I could reason to myself, *Why waste a good workout by pigging out*?

Lo and behold, it worked. It took several months for the motivation to kick in, but I found myself finally putting the healthy eating and exercise back to back. My weight still fluctuated to a certain extent, but a return to obesity was the last thing on my mind.

Fast forward a few years. I was married with two little kids and beginning a new career. Talk about transitions! The excess weight started creeping back on like an obnoxious neighbor knocking on the door after an extended vacation. Those old behaviors, which I thought were buried in the past, dug themselves out of the dirt and hopped back on to my plate. Even though I tried to fool myself into thinking they just reappeared out of nowhere, I was the one who picked up the shovel, led the excavation, and resuscitated them with a vengeance.

This time, however, my overeating had really escalated. So I turned to the formula that had worked before. Why not? It worked then. Why wouldn't it work now? I started working out. Exercise would be the trick.

I joined the Sergeants Fitness Program, waking up before sunrise to be yelled into shape by a bunch of former marines. It did wonders for my biceps, but little for my waistline. I was more diligent with pizza than pushups.

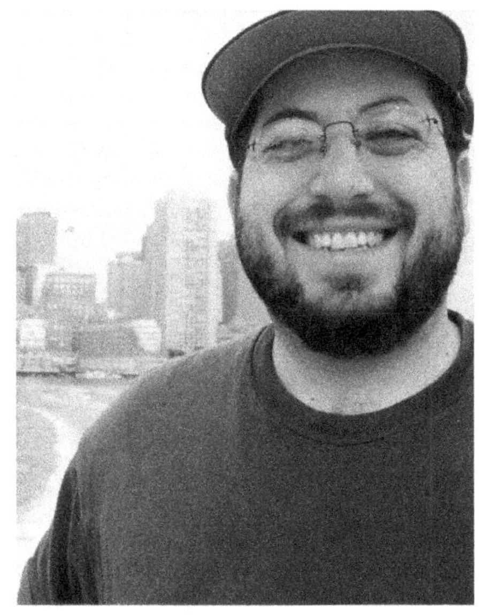

I fiddled with fad diets, endured half-day fasts, and dabbled with diet pills. The stimulants didn't magically make me lose weight; I just ate faster.

I joined an expensive health club and worked out religiously. When that didn't make a dent in my bulge, I started hiring a personal trainer. My inner core was in great shape. But you wouldn't know it because it was covered with layers of flab. I exercised incessantly and still weighed 300 pounds.

I was disgusted and humiliated. Why wasn't it working? Why wasn't the exercise motivating me to stay away from the fast food, to refrain from running to restaurants and to make healthy and normal food choices like it did when I was younger?

I didn't have the disposable income to throw at fancy gym membership and personal trainers – let alone the cost of continually eating out. The added expense added to my frustration. I was stuck in a spiraling cycle of self-loathing.

I had come to a demoralizing conclusion: maybe I was destined to be fat. Why bother fighting it anymore? Maybe lots and lots was my lot in life.

Enough! I didn't care anymore.

I was at my bottom. The clarity and conviction I had in other aspects of my life completely escaped me when it came to food. Discipline and determination disappeared down a donut hole. My "Saturday night" behavior, my late-night gorging and eating to excess were habits against which I felt I had no control.

As hard and as often as I tried, I just could not win the war. Completely desperate and humiliated, I finally acknowledged that I had to stop working on dieting and start working on changing myself.

Thus began my trek toward transformation.

It hit me, of all places, in the dressing room of a Target department store. It was early August, 2002. In a few days I would be taking a trans-Atlantic flight and I simply couldn't stomach the thought of sitting so long in what was for me a very cramped airplane seat, with slacks that were popping at the seams and wearing out in all the wrong places.

For years I was convinced I would lose the weight and therefore rarely bought clothes that actually fit my current girth. I deluded myself into thinking that I could buy the size I thought I should be in, and that would induce me to slim down into them. It never worked. As my weight gained over time, my wardrobe was usually one size behind.

This time, however, I said uncle and found a pair of size 44 pants. I was a 34 waist for my wedding eight years earlier and had been busting out of 42s for the past few hard-headed years before taking the fateful trip to Target.

There I was, sitting on the bench in the dressing room staring at a pair of $30 khakis. I held them up, one hand on either end of the waist band, spreading my arms wider and wider apart, amazed at how much fabric it took to wrap around my rotund rear end. I kept staring and staring. I wasn't angry or resentful. There was no disgust or self-ridicule. Rather, a calming wave of acceptance and purpose engulfed me – serenity and certainty at the same time. It wasn't about trying to find the newest diet or most rigid workout routine. I had been there and done all that.

Sitting there with the slacks in my hands, I felt the vast separation between my head and heart finally come together. For the previous half year, I had intellectually realized that I needed to make a wholesale change in myself, in my coping mechanisms with life and obsession with self-indulgence. Despite all the time, money and energy – all the sweat equity I invested in building up a sweat--I was intimidated to really go "all in." That was the irony of it all. I went to great lengths not to go to ANY lengths necessary.

I was grasping at external solutions for an internal problem. That's why I could never get a grip. I hung on to the last rays of hope that I could somehow find the magic formula, or quick fix to change my body instead of changing myself.

I had a palpable fear of feeling restricted and deprived. I was enslaved by my entitlement to indulge. Saying "no" to my urge to eat felt like a colossal confrontation against which I cowered to contest. I was handicapped by my irrationality, living in the lie that only with excess food would I be sufficiently satisfied.

On an otherwise ordinary summer day, however, I accepted the challenge of unconditional honesty. I felt at ease and emotionally prepared to do whatever it took to CHANGE my relationship with food, not just to try and lose weight. I was ready to say "no."

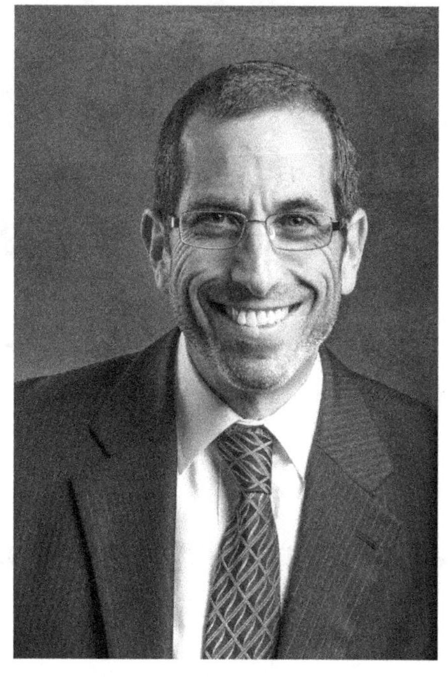

For goodness sake, I was having an epiphany in the dressing room of a Target department store. Enough was finally enough.

"Thank you for your life-changing information and inspiration."

- Aron, Atlanta, Georgia

3

A FOOD PLAN

A LIGHTNING BOLT SHOWS DIRECTION, BUT WE HAVE TO TAKE THE STEPS

You're stranded in the middle of a desert on a freezing, pitch-black winter night with no clue which way to return to civilization. Your frostbite is overcome only by your fear.

All of a sudden, a bolt of lightning crashes to the ground with a thundering clap some distance over your right shoulder, illuminating an oasis and surrounding village. Even though it lasts for less than a second, you now know which way to go. You're thrilled and relieved. But you're not waiting for another bolt from the sky to pick you up like a mystical chariot and carry you home. All it did was show you direction. Now, you have to take the steps.

So often in life, so many of us are waiting for the miracle to change us or to change our circumstances. We're much more likely to get struck by that lightning bolt than to win the lottery of life – where everything instantaneously changes from bad to good – from hard to easy.

I think the essence of my epiphany in the dressing room was just that. I finally understood that I had to start taking the steps to change my relationship with food, and no longer just hang out at the corner waiting for the magic weight-loss bus to arrive. I must have had the wrong schedule, because it never came.

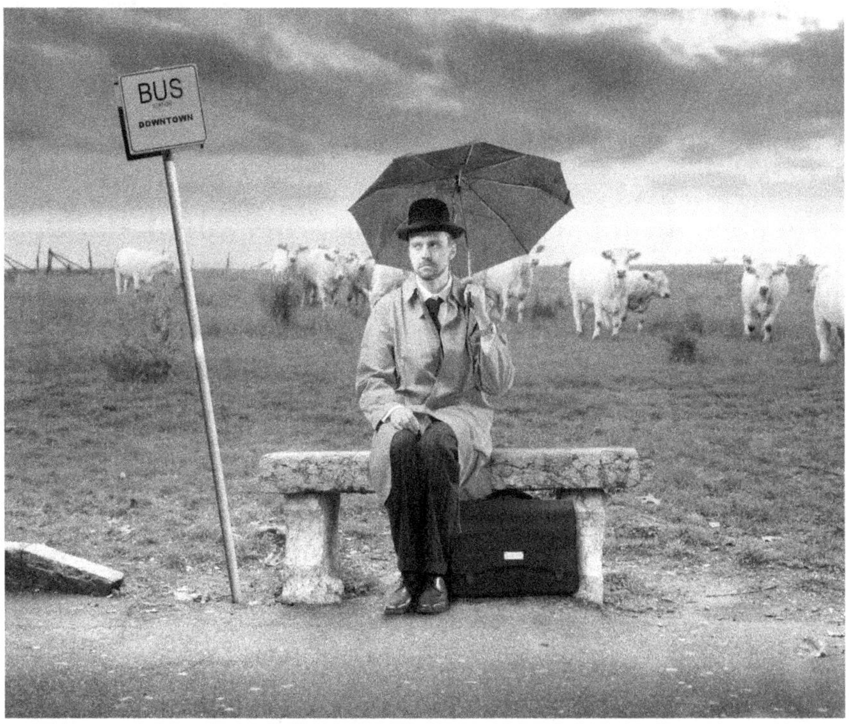

I also had to be willing to wholeheartedly accept suggestions, direction, and advice from a mentor and a community of people who had their share of success and were willing to share it with me (see the chapter C.H.A.N.G.E. about Humility and Accountability). And most of all, I needed a plan of action to help me navigate my day without hurting myself with food, but rather to nourish, sustain, and energize.

I needed a food plan.

"If you fail to plan, then you are planning to fail."
- Benjamin Franklin

A plan of action with distinct directions, guidelines, and boundaries is critical to achieving any meaningful goal in life. This is even more crucial when it comes to successful weight loss.

So why is it that so many diet programs paint pristine pictures of promise, but fail to color in the intricate details? Because there is a widely held misconception that we can somehow navigate to the finish line on our own. We're bombarded with the hottest craze, latest theory, or newest discovery of a miraculous fat-burning plant from South America but are left to magically access our innate intuition and self-awareness to make the right decisions at the right times, to conquer our cravings and appease our appetite.

This approach may indeed work for other areas of our life. Our instincts, insights, and acumen might make us accomplished and effective parents, educators, managers, or consultants. They could be real assets for us in business and at home. But it's not a formula for success when it comes to food--at least not if we're one of the millions of people perpetually plummeting up and down the dieting roller coaster.

In short: *Intuitive eating doesn't work.* Our intuition is broken when it comes to food. It's not an asset, it's a liability.

Now, does that make us a bad person? Of course not. Just like there's no personality defect or character flaw for those of us who are visually impaired and need to use corrective lenses in order to see straight. We're ready, willing, and able to access an external resource to compensate for an internal deficiency--to repeatedly pick up a tool to correct our visual misalignment. They're called glasses.

And so it is with eating. Our vision is always askew when it comes to food. That's why our weight-loss journeys have invariably ended up in the ditch of dieting on the side of the road. What looked like smooth sailing and comfortable coasting quickly became a huge pot hole and dangerous detour that we failed to circumvent in time. Crash and burn--or in our case, crash and binge. Again and again.

That's why a well-defined food plan – with crystal-clear guidelines, boundaries and directions--is crucial. It provides the proper prescription for us to see clearly in any situation, to steer through the myriad of challenging food environments that have incessantly tripped us up in the past.

The food plan is the corrective lenses that allows us to successfully travel toward our weight-loss destination, avoiding the hazards and pitfalls that have littered our path up to this point.

FEELINGS ARE NOT ALWAYS FACTS

To understand why a food plan is an essential element for developing and maintaining a healthy relationship with eating, we have to learn the difference between *hunger* and *appetite*. For this purpose, I use the following definitions:

Hunger is our body's need for proper nutrition.

Appetite is our spontaneous desire to use food for physical enjoyment, indulgence, comfort, or any other perceived momentary benefit, the most common being stress relief or emotional eating. Sound familiar?

More often than not, we end up eating based on how we feel at that moment, as opposed to what our body truly needs – either overeating healthy foods because they taste good, or impulsively making unhealthy choices.

The physical sensations generated by hunger and appetite are strikingly similar. We all know what it's like to have hunger pangs, cravings, and temptations. But what we've done so frequently in the past is conclude that just because we're feeling this way, it must mean we need to eat. We misdiagnose what is really going on in our body.

We'll often panic at those first feelings and grab whatever's nearby.

And that's why a personalized, healthy, and robust food plan is so important. It takes the guesswork out of it and guides us through the day, delineating from which food groups we should choose, how much, and when. It's our customized GPS, mapping out each leg of our daily eating excursion. Without it, we're lost. It doesn't dissolve our feelings or solve our problems. But it does give us a clear path and direction for how not to eat over them.

A proper food plan is not about crash dieting. It's not about drastically restricting calories or cutting out necessary food groups in order to "kick start" our weight loss. It's about providing us with the framework to have a healthy and sustainable relationship with food – which is the bedrock for the Soveya Solution.

And guess what? If we do that, we'll actually lose *more* weight over a longer period of time – and even more importantly, we'll develop the skills and behavior to *maintain* a healthy body size for the rest of our life. I'm living proof. I lost the bulk of my weight – 110 pounds – in 11 months, without crash dieting.

Q.Q.T. – QUALITY – QUANTITY – TIMING

Okay, now that we've established that our goal is not to focus on losing weight, but on developing a healthy relationship with food, we have to define our terms. And that begins with intellectually acknowledging and emotionally accepting its objective function. Not what we *want* it to be, or what role we *feel* it should fulfill in our life.

But what's the true and genuine purpose of food? Why do we need to eat?

It's pretty simple and straightforward. The function of food is to fuel our body.

Let's begin with a basic biology lesson. The human body is made up of trillions of cells, which serve as the fundamental building blocks of life. These cells need to be nourished to survive and thrive. They require a daily absorption of six essential nutrients: protein, carbohydrates, lipids (fat), vitamins, minerals, water.

They are called essential for two reasons: 1, we can't live without them; 2, we don't produce them on our own, we need to get them from an external source. That source is food.

If a person doesn't have food and water, they'll die. We unquestionably recognize that eating is the singular most important thing we do to keep us alive. That's its function, to provide us with health, energy, and vitality.

But the tricky part is that we have to make that choice. It doesn't happen on its own. Proper rest is also critically important for health and wellness. However, the body, barring any outside interference, will cause itself to sleep.

Many of us have probably experienced some sort of extreme fatigue when we just couldn't stand up anymore. Our body is screaming at us to rest, and as long as we allow the process to happen, we will replenish our energy through sufficient sleep.

Nourishment is not the same. It's not a passive behavior. Our body can scream at us to eat, but if we don't take a proactive role, it can't do it on its own. It can't feed itself. Therefore, at the most primary level, we eat to live, to give fuel to our body like we fuel our car.

And the three criteria for proper fueling are classified as Q.Q.T. – Quality, Quantity, Timing – the proper quality of fuel, the right quantity, at the right time.

Take the following example: As you're heading to the gas station, you see what looks like a typical lemonade stand at the corner of the block. But as you pull closer, you notice they're not advertising lemonade, but gasoline – at 39¢ per gallon, no less. You're definitely intrigued, since gas at the pump is going to set you back close to $3 per gallon.

But it's only going to take you one or two seconds to decide to continue driving to the nearest station and shell out almost ten times more. Why? Because at this "lemonade stand" you have no idea what they're going to put in your tank. It could be lemonade, sugar, water, who knows. You're willing to pay the much higher price because you understand that your car needs the right *quality* of fuel for it to function properly and not break down.

Okay, now that you're at the pump, how much gas are you going to put in? Probably between 14-16 gallons, if you're on empty. You're not going to put in two gallons and then drive off, because then you'd have to stop at another station every half hour. And you're not going to willfully overflow your tank, or once it's full, take the nozzle and spray gas over your hood or windshield for the thrill of it. That'd be pretty silly, expensive, and smelly – ever try and get the stench of gasoline out of your clothes?

Why won't you do that? Because you know that you need the right *quantity* of fuel that your car commands – not too little and not too much – but the accurate amount it requires at that moment.

Which brings us to the *timing*. When you're on the highway and the low-fuel light starts flashing, you'll probably stop at the next service area. Even though you may be tempted to try and drive on fumes until you get home, or find a place with a cheaper price, the thought of being stranded on the side of the interstate waiting hours for the tow truck to show up with a gas can is not so appealing.

You're responsible enough to fuel your car at the right times, *before* things become too compromised.

I'm guessing we have all have mastered the proficiency of Q.Q.T. when it comes to our vehicle. After all, it's not rocket science.

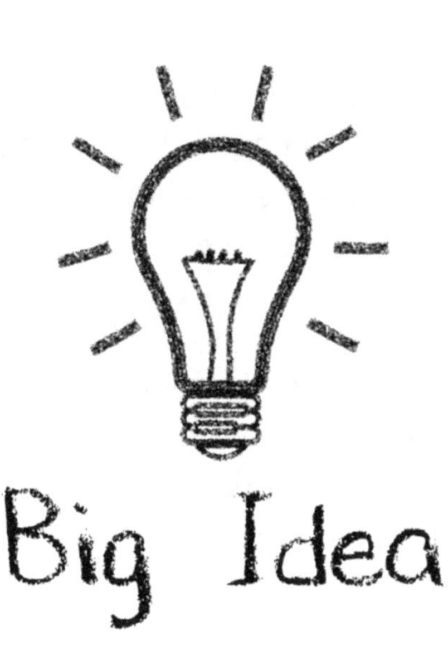

Now, we have to transfer that skill set to our eating--because ensuring the right quality of foods, the correct quantity and at the ideal times of day is critical for fueling the engine of our body.

That's where a responsible and robust food plan comes in. It's designed to meticulously manage our daily quality, quantity, and timing by:

- Maximizing the nutritional value of your choices and minimizing refined carbohydrates and empty calories
- Stabilizing portion control, substantially nourishing your healthy cells while starving your unhealthy fat cells, resulting in *conscientious* and consistent weight loss
- Establishing an ideal metabolic rate, steady blood-sugar level, and providing continual energy throughout the day
- Detoxing the body from addictive substances and

curtailing compulsive behaviors (impulsive eating and spontaneous choices)

A customized food plan is designed to meet the unique needs of each individual based on several criteria such as: height, weight, age, gender, current health and medical status (such as pregnant, nursing, diabetic, hypoglycemic), activity level, daily schedule, and occupational demands. For instance, a nurse pulling a 7 p.m. – 7 a.m. shift is going to necessitate a different food plan structure than an accountant working 9 a.m. – 5 p.m.

The baseline requirements for everyone begin uniformly with protein, grains, vegetables, and fruit, and are then adapted into a suggested daily meal schedule with the recommended quantities delineated for each category. I always emphasize that whatever a client's end-result meal plan looks like, I strongly encourage them to share it with their health-care professionals for review. Best nutrition practices are best played as a team sport. The accompanying Smith siblings' samplings illustrate possible permutations of the Soveya plan. You can go to our website, *soveya.com*, for more information about our programs and how to obtain a personalized food plan.

CUSTOMIZED FOOD PLAN FOR

JANE SMITH

SOVEYA
WEIGHT-LOSS SOLUTION

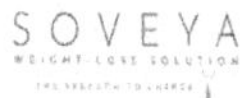

MEALS

BREAKFAST
PROTEIN - GRAIN
MORNING SNACK
1/2 PROTEIN - FRUIT
LUNCH
PROTEIN - VEGETABLE - FAT
DINNER
PROTEIN - GRAIN - VEGETABLE - FAT - FRUIT

GUIDELINES:

(1) Wait 4 -6 hours between meals; 2 -3 hours with planned snacks
(2) No eating between meals and/or planned snacks
(3) Drink up to 64 oz of water a day; flavored but unsweetened seltzer; tea; coffee (skim milk ideal; low-fat if needed)
(4) Use the following freely: spices; lemon juice; mustard; cooking spray; vinegar; unsweetened soy sauce; liquid aminos

GOALS (Q.Q.T. - Quality, Quantity, Timing):

(1) Maximize nutritional value of choices (robust calories vs. empty calories)
(2) Stabilize and regulate portion control & timing of meals
(3) Minimize refined carbohydrates such as flour products (cakes; cookies; pasta; most bread products) and added sweeteners – natural or artificial (cane or beet sugar; HFCS; honey; splenda; sorbitol; aspartame; stevia; truvia; agave nectar; nutrasweet; maltodextrin; barley malt; mannitol; fructose)
(4) Establish steady Metabolic rate and blood-sugar levels; maintain consistent energy; detox body from addictive substances that trigger cravings
(5) Eliminate compulsive behaviors (impulsive eating and spontaneous choices)

PROTEINS

12 oz low-fat milk or unsweetened soy milk
8 oz plain yogurt
6 oz soft cheese: cottage; ricotta; feta; farmers
4 oz meat: chicken; turkey; fish; chick peas; beans; tofu; edamame
2 oz sliced cheese; 2 cheese sticks
2 oz nuts or nut butter (e.g. peanuts; almonds; cashews; walnuts; unsweetened peanut butter; unsweetened almond butter)
2 whole eggs (or 4 egg whites)

GRAINS (breakfast cereals weigh dry before cooking; all others weigh after)
2 oz HOT CEREAL (dry weight): oatmeal (not instant); oat bran; cream of wheat; farina; wheat germ; grits; quinoa flakes
2 oz COLD CEREAL (dry weight):
* Group A (maximize this choice): made from whole grain, not refined flour & has 0 grams of added sugar.
* Group B (minimize this choice): made from refined flour & has *no more than* 5 grams of added sugar per serving.
* Group C (avoid this choice): made from refined flour & has *more than* 5 grams of added sugar per serving.
4 oz COOKED GRAIN: whole-grain rice (brown, jasmine, basmati); potatoes (sweet, red, white); kasha; barley; quinoa; bulgur, farro, millet, amaranth
4 large rice cakes or 6 medium rice cakes or corn thins

VEGETABLES: (12 oz - cooked or raw)
FRUITS: (1 average size whole fruit; or 6 oz cut-up fruit; or 2 oz dried fruit)
FATS (1 tablespoon unsaturated) examples: olive oil; sesame oil; flax seed oil; canola oil; safflower/sunflower oil; peanut oil; whole mayo; techina;

For illustration purposes only

CUSTOMIZED FOOD PLAN FOR

JILL SMITH

SOVEYA
WEIGHT-LOSS SOLUTION

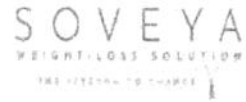

MEALS

BREAKFAST
PROTEIN - GRAIN - FRUIT
LUNCH
PROTEIN - GRAIN - VEGETABLE - FAT
AFTERNOON SNACK
1/2 PROTEIN - FRUIT
DINNER
PROTEIN - VEGETABLE - FAT - FRUIT

GUIDELINES:

(1) Wait 4 -6 hours between meals; 2 -3 hours with planned snacks
(2) No eating between meals and/or planned snacks
(3) Drink up to 64 oz of water a day; flavored but unsweetened seltzer; tea; coffee (skim milk ideal; low-fat if needed)
(4) Use the following freely: spices; lemon juice; mustard; cooking spray; vinegar; unsweetened soy sauce; liquid aminos

GOALS (Q.Q.T. - Quality, Quantity, Timing):

(1) Maximize nutritional value of choices (robust calories vs. empty calories)
(2) Stabilize and regulate portion control & timing of meals
(3) Minimize refined carbohydrates such as flour products (cakes; cookies; pasta; most bread products) and added sweeteners – natural or artificial (cane or beet sugar; HFCS; honey; splenda; sorbitol; aspartame; stevia; truvia; agave nectar; nutrasweet; maltodextrin; barley malt; mannitol; fructose)
(4) Establish steady Metabolic rate and blood-sugar levels; maintain consistent energy; detox body from addictive substances that trigger cravings
(5) Eliminate compulsive behaviors (impulsive eating and spontaneous choices)

PROTEINS

10 oz low-fat milk or unsweetened soy milk
6 oz plain yogurt
4 oz soft cheese: cottage; ricotta; feta; farmers
4 oz meat; chicken; turkey; fish; chick peas; beans; tofu; edamame
2 oz sliced cheese; 2 cheese sticks
2 oz nuts or nut butter (e.g. peanuts; almonds; cashews; walnuts; unsweetened peanut butter; unsweetened almond butter)
2 whole eggs (or 4 egg whites)

GRAINS (breakfast cereals weigh dry before cooking; all others weigh after)
1 oz HOT CEREAL (dry weight): oatmeal (not instant); oat bran; cream of wheat; farina; wheat germ; grits; quinoa flakes
1 oz COLD CEREAL (dry weight):
* Group A (maximize this choice): made from whole grain, not refined flour & has 0 grams of added sugar.
* Group B (minimize this choice): made from refined flour & has *no more than* 5 grams of added sugar per serving.
* Group C (avoid this choice): made from refined flour & has *more than* 5 grams of added sugar per serving.
3 oz COOKED GRAIN: whole-grain rice (brown, jasmine, basmati); potatoes (sweet, red, white); kasha; barley; quinoa; bulgur, farro, millet, amaranth
2 large rice cakes or 4 medium rice cakes or corn thins

VEGETABLES: (10 oz - cooked or raw)
FRUITS: (1 average size whole fruit; or 6 oz cut-up fruit; or 2 oz dried fruit)
FATS (1 tablespoon unsaturated) examples: olive oil; sesame oil; flax seed oil; canola oil; safflower/sunflower oil; peanut oil; whole mayo; techina;

For illustration purposes only

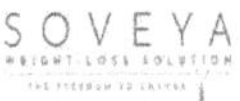

CUSTOMIZED FOOD PLAN FOR
JOE SMITH

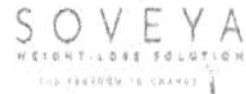

MEALS

BREAKFAST
PROTEIN - GRAIN - FRUIT
MORNING SNACK
1/2 PROTEIN - FRUIT
LUNCH
PROTEIN - GRAIN - VEGETABLE - FAT - FRUIT
DINNER
PROTEIN - GRAIN - VEGETABLE - FAT

GUIDELINES:

(1) Wait 4 -6 hours between meals; 2 -3 hours with planned snacks
(2) No eating between meals and/or planned snacks
(3) Drink up to 64 oz of water a day; flavored but unsweetened seltzer; tea; coffee (skim milk ideal; low-fat if needed)
(4) Use the following freely: spices; lemon juice; mustard; cooking spray; vinegar; unsweetened soy sauce; liquid aminos

GOALS (Q.Q.T. - Quality, Quantity, Timing):

(1) Maximize nutritional value of choices (robust calories vs. empty calories)
(2) Stabilize and regulate portion control & timing of meals
(3) Minimize refined carbohydrates such as flour products (cakes; cookies; pasta; most bread products) and added sweeteners - natural or artificial (cane or beet sugar; HFCS; honey; splenda; sorbitol; aspartame; stevia; truvia; agave nectar; nutrasweet; maltodextrin; barley malt; mannitol; fructose)
(4) Establish steady Metabolic rate and blood-sugar levels; maintain consistent energy; detox body from addictive substances that trigger cravings
(5) Eliminate compulsive behaviors (impulsive eating and spontaneous choices)

PROTEINS

12 oz low-fat milk or unsweetened soy milk
8 oz plain yogurt
6 oz soft cheese: cottage; ricotta; feta; farmers
6 oz meat; chicken; turkey; fish; chick peas; beans; tofu; edamame
3 oz sliced cheese; 3 cheese sticks
3 oz nuts or nut butter (e.g. peanuts; almonds; cashews; walnuts; unsweetened peanut butter; unsweetened almond butter)
3 whole eggs (or 6 egg whites)

GRAINS (breakfast cereals weigh dry before cooking; all others weigh after)

2 oz HOT CEREAL (dry weight): oatmeal (not instant); oat bran; cream of wheat; farina; wheat germ; grits; quinoa flakes
2 oz COLD CEREAL (dry weight):
* Group A (maximize this choice): made from whole grain, not refined flour & has 0 grams of added sugar.
* Group B (minimize this choice): made from refined flour & has *no more than* 5 grams of added sugar per serving.
* Group C (avoid this choice): made from refined flour & has *more than* 5 grams of added sugar per serving.
5 oz COOKED GRAIN: whole-grain rice (brown, jasmine, basmati); potatoes (sweet, red, white); kasha; barley; quinoa; bulgur, farro, millet, amaranth
4 large rice cakes or 6 medium rice cakes or corn thins

VEGETABLES: (14 oz - cooked or raw)
FRUITS: (1 average size whole fruit; or 6 oz cut-up fruit; or 2 oz dried fruit)
FATS (2 tablespoons unsaturated) examples: olive oil; sesame oil; flax seed oil; canola oil; safflower/sunflower oil; peanut oil; whole mayo; techina;

For illustration purposes only

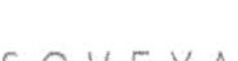

CUSTOMIZED FOOD PLAN FOR
JOHN SMITH

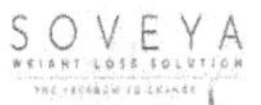

MEALS

BREAKFAST
PROTEIN - GRAIN - FRUIT

LUNCH
PROTEIN - VEGETABLE - FAT - FRUIT

DINNER
PROTEIN - GRAIN - VEGETABLE - FAT - FRUIT

GUIDELINES:

(1) Wait 4 -6 hours between meals
(2) No eating between meals
(3) Drink up to 64 oz of water a day; flavored but unsweetened seltzer; tea; coffee (skim milk ideal; low-fat if needed)
(4) Use the following freely: spices; lemon juice; mustard; cooking spray; vinegar; unsweetened soy sauce; liquid aminos

GOALS (Q.Q.T. - Quality, Quantity, Timing):

(1) Maximize nutritional value of choices (robust calories vs. empty calories)
(2) Stabilize and regulate portion control & timing of meals
(3) Minimize refined carbohydrates such as flour products (cakes; cookies; pasta; most bread products) and added sweeteners - natural or artificial (cane or beet sugar; HFCS; honey; splenda; sorbitol; aspartame; stevia; truvia; agave nectar; nutrasweet; maltodextrin; barley malt; mannitol; fructose)
(4) Establish steady Metabolic rate and blood-sugar levels; maintain consistent energy; detox body from addictive substances that trigger cravings
(5) Eliminate compulsive behaviors (impulsive eating and spontaneous choices)

PROTEINS

12 oz low-fat milk or unsweetened soy milk
8 oz plain yogurt
6 oz soft cheese: cottage; ricotta; feta; farmers
6 oz meat; chicken; turkey; fish; chick peas; beans; tofu; edamame
3 oz sliced cheese; 3 cheese sticks
3 oz nuts or nut butter (e.g. peanuts; almonds; cashews; walnuts; unsweetened peanut butter; unsweetened almond butter)
3 whole eggs (or 6 egg whites)

GRAINS (breakfast cereals weigh dry before cooking; all others weigh after)

3 oz HOT CEREAL (dry weight): oatmeal (not instant); oat bran; cream of wheat; farina; wheat germ; grits; quinoa flakes
3 oz COLD CEREAL (dry weight):
* Group A (maximize this choice): made from whole grain, not refined flour & has 0 grams of added sugar.
* Group B (minimize this choice): made from refined flour & has *no more than* 5 grams of added sugar per serving.
* Group C (avoid this choice): made from refined flour & has *more than* 5 grams of added sugar per serving.
6 oz COOKED GRAIN: whole-grain rice (brown, jasmine, basmati); potatoes (sweet, red, white); kasha; barley; quinoa; bulgur, farro, millet, amaranth
4 large rice cakes or 6 medium rice cakes or corn thins

VEGETABLES: (16 oz - cooked or raw)
FRUITS: (1 average size whole fruit; or 6 oz cut-up fruit; or 2 oz dried fruit)
FATS (2 tablespoons unsaturated) examples: olive oil; sesame oil; flax seed oil; canola oil; safflower/sunflower oil; peanut oil; whole mayo; techina;

For illustration purposes only

FUNCTION VS. BENEFIT

Okay, everything seems sound and sensible up to this point. But there is ostensibly one huge flaw in our analogy. A car doesn't have any sensation when the gas goes in, other than moving the dial on our dashboard from left to right.

But food tastes *really* good! Eating something we enjoy is a stimulating physical sensation, creating a fun, comforting and/or indulgent experience.

Is that necessarily a bad thing? Not at all! We have taste buds for a reason – to enjoy the act of fueling our body. What a gift. What a benefit.

What a challenge!

And that's why it's essential to distinguish between hunger vs. appetite – and function vs. benefit. The function of eating is not for a temporary pleasure. It's to fuel our body for energy and vitality. And while we do that responsibly, it can be – and should be – an enjoyable experience.

Function should not *rule out* fun, it should *rule over* fun. The pleasure of eating is a wonderful benefit, but not its underlying purpose.

Six-year-old Miriam is playing outside with her friends on a beautiful summer evening. She hears her mother call, "Mimi, it's time to come in now for dinner." Is her first instinct, "Sure Mom, right away!"

Probably not. Why? Because Miriam is in the midst of a fun activity and she wants to perpetuate that enjoyable experience. That's a perfectly healthy and normal response. But it doesn't necessarily mean it's the right thing for her to do. Just because she feels that way for the moment doesn't make it the appropriate action to take.

Feelings aren't always facts.

Left to her own momentary impulses, she'll forgo the responsible choice to extend her entertainment, and in the process will miss dinner, go to sleep late, and be cranky and less productive the next day. In the end, the cost will far outweigh the benefit.

I'm not at all suggesting that Miriam should never play and have a good time with her friends. What I'm illustrating is that she needs external direction to help her do it within the proper boundaries.

See where we're going here?

"Eli, you lost 130 pounds and kept it off for all these years--what changed in you?" This is one of the most common questions I get.

My answer is always the same. It wasn't about being strong or being strict, or some new found willpower to conquer my cravings. It was all about my willingness to confront the challenge of unconditional (and often uncomfortable) honesty, and self-maturation. To stop rationalizing and justifying my immediate desire to indulge, and to be willing to grow up – and grow out of the "six-year-old syndrome" – that just because I felt that I wanted to eat, didn't necessarily mean that was the right choice for me to make at that moment.

A healthy, robust food plan with well-defined guidelines and goals was one of the lynchpins of my transformation. The food plan gave me the 20/20 vision to navigate my way through my daily nutrition, helping me differentiate between feelings and facts, between hunger and appetite.

And here's the secret (even though I incessantly implore that there are no secrets, shortcuts or magic pills when it comes to healthy and sustainable weight loss). Are you ready? The *stronger* the boundaries are of our plan, the *easier* it will be for us, and the *greater success* we'll have.

Why? Because the less guesswork and impulsivity we allow, the greater our ability to choose facts over feelings, to satisfy our hunger instead of indulging our appetite. Eating to meet our body's needs has measurable limits, but feeding our feelings is often a bottomless pit.

There's nothing wrong with prioritizing *our* needs in the face of all our other taxing demands (see the chapter <u>C.H.A.N.G.E.</u> about the attitude of Necessity). In fact, it's the responsible thing to do. It's critically important for our success. Why? Because no one else is going to do it for us!

We begin the day with a precisely prescribed and

personalized plan of action, charting out the proper food groups for each meal, with apt and accurate quantities scheduled for the ideal times. Whether we're overwhelmed, overworked, stressed, or fatigued, our food plan will be the bedrock of consistency and accountability, where we would otherwise be much more susceptible to spontaneously succumb to sudden temptation.

A concrete commitment first thing in the morning to diligently stick within the parameters of our plan – and not allow any wiggle room no matter what circumstances or triggers may come our way – will give us a tremendous freedom from food obsession (see the chapter Clarity is Key about the Clarity List). After each meal, we'll know that all of our nutritional needs will have been met, and that we will be satiated, satisfied, and energized to go on with our day. We'll learn to live life between meals without the ever-present possibility of noshing, grazing, or grabbing.

EAT TO YOUR FILL, NOT TILL YOU'RE FULL

For many of us, satiation is a learned skill, not necessarily a naturally occurring feeling. Our "cutoff switch" is either broken or delayed. The reason is because we're shooting for the wrong target – we're eating to fill our stomach instead of fueling our cells. The function of digestion and metabolism is to distribute these essential nutrients to the trillions of cells in our body – which results in extended satiation and consistent energy and vitality for the next several hours of our day.

Our stomach is an incredibly powerful agitator (kind of like a washing machine), breaking down the food from a solid to a liquid so it can be absorbed in our small intestine and continue the path of being metabolized in our body. But it's just a processing plant, as it were – not the final destination.

And this process can take up to 60 minutes to fully complete. That's why our grandmothers warned us against going swimming within an hour of eating. We would interrupt the digestive progression and cause cramps because the food hadn't been thoroughly digested.

The initial sensations of satiation can begin around 5 -10 minutes after we start eating, but the complete satisfaction takes a little more time. We have to respect this process and be patient for those first few moments.

However, if we stuff down our meal with the intention of stopping only after feeling our stomachs are stuffed and distended, we have, by definition, overeaten, because all that excess food still needs to be digested and distributed, causing us to consume hundreds more calories than needed and resulting in that bloating and discomfort we've experienced so often.

That was my modus operandi. I lived for – or more aptly, was killing myself for that "full" feeling. So, at thirty-eight years old, for the first time in my life, I had to be willing to be uncomfortable with wanting more food, yet not eating. I had to be willing to learn how to nourish myself instead of indulging myself. Now that was stepping outside of my comfort zone.

I had to train my body to get used to the appropriate amounts of food, which meant eating less meat and potatoes than I had been previously, and more vegetables and fruit. It's not what I felt like doing, but what I needed to do.

For the first few weeks, it was distressing for me to eat six ounces of steak instead of sixteen and certainly out of character to make sure I had a sufficient serving of vegetables for lunch and dinner. But I was learning to be comfortable being uncomfortable.

Why did I want to do that? I'm certainly not a masochist. Because the discomfort of being morbidly obese was exponentially worse than the temporary discomfort of adjusting to appropriate eating habits. I had to take the pain to the make the gain – or in this case, lose the weight.

And breakfast. I was actually eating breakfast. Every day. That was the biggest miracle of all. I woke up with an appetite each morning instead of bloated and distended. I enjoyed my meals and stuck to a consistent schedule: breakfast no later than 9 a.m., then lunch and dinner at four- to six-hour intervals.

If the compulsion for binging at night started creeping in, I followed a "radical" suggestion – I went to bed. If it's a hard day, make it a short day. It wasn't rocket science.

It was nutrition 101. But for me, it was my doctoral thesis in healthy living.

It wasn't so easy to fit consistent meal times into my hectic schedule. I often had professional events at night and appointments first thing in the morning. But I made it work. I made my food plan the most important priority of my day.

Business meetings over lunch were rather awkward at first, especially when I was leading the proceedings. When everyone else had downed their sandwich and bag of chips in the first five minutes, I was still working on my salad, vegetables, and piece of protein twenty minutes later.

Did I feel awkward and a little self-conscious? Sure. Would I rather remain at 300 pounds and fit in with sandwich crowd, or do what I needed to do to live in a normal-sized body? Thankfully, I was willing to take the pain to make the gain. And I've never had any regrets since.

This was my first step toward true transformation and experiencing the incredible freedom to change – and starting to really understand that nothing tastes as good as feeling good feels.

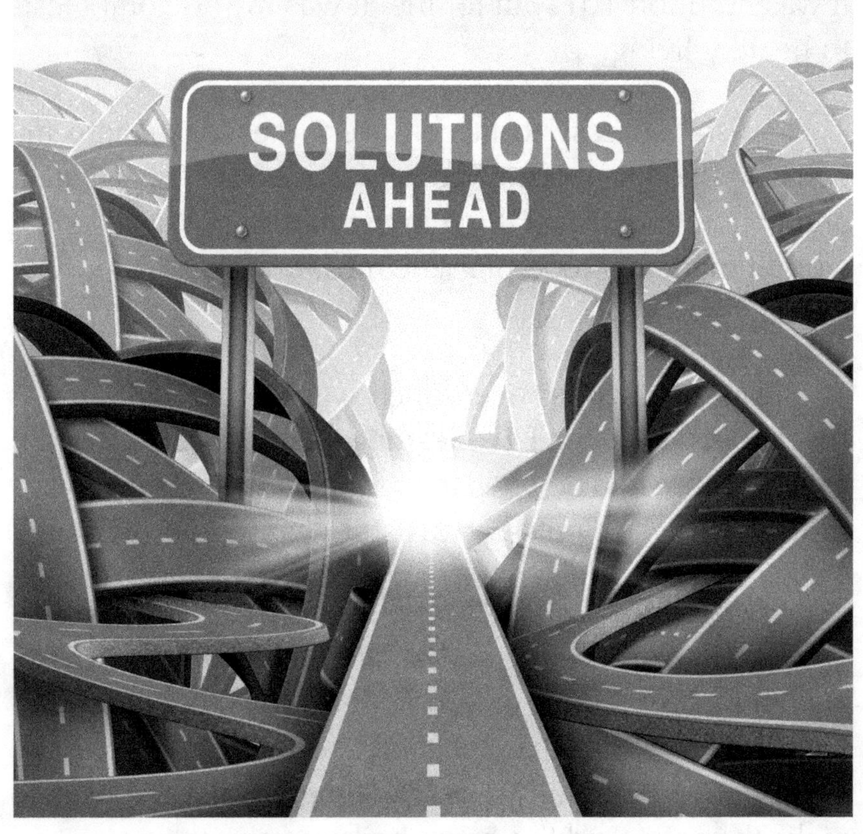

4

STAY INSIDE THE BLUE BOX

DON'T FEED YOUR FEELINGS

As I mentioned earlier, one of the primary goals of the Soveya Food Plan is to help the body detoxify from addictive substances as well as curtail compulsive behaviors with food, such as impulsive eating and making spontaneous choices. You might have glossed over that part or not given it much thought.

Trust me, it's a very weighty subject.

I believe that compulsive eating is arguably the most common, yet least acknowledged addictive behavior. A very general and succinct synopsis of addiction could be summarized as: a repetitive behavior with destruct consequences and an inability to stop on your own.

Addiction can be to either a substance, such as alcohol or narcotics, or to a process and activity such as gambling. In both circumstances, the pleasure chemicals of endorphins and dopamine are released from the brain, creating an insatiable desire for more.

THE CASUAL DRINKER VS. THE ALCOHOLIC

What's the difference between the two? A casual drinker can take one drink then stop on their own. They can manage to internally place a boundary around that behavior. For an alcoholic, it's like being tethered to a freight train. Once it starts moving, it feels impossible to stop. Upon taking that first drink, it's as if they're powerless over that second drink.

Even though the casual drinker and the alcoholic both get a buzz from the booze, the body of the casual drinker metabolizes the alcohol much more quickly and efficiently, whereas the brain of the alcoholic reacts much more intensely – roughly like an acute sensitivity and allergic reaction. It creates a compulsive desire to replicate that feeling, hence increasing one's threshold and tolerance and requiring more of that substance to elicit the same response. That intense reward system and cycle of behavior can also be triggered by other drugs and activities.

So what in the world does this have to do with eating? Everything.

I posit that compulsive eating comprises both an addiction to a substance and to a process – the dastardly daily double. Sugar (and really, any refined carbohydrate) is the substance, and the bingeing behavior of eating for comfort and indulgence, to alleviate stress or to anesthetize ourselves from emotional anxiety is the process.

Let's start with the substance.

Upon digestion, the body begins to metabolize all food – from celery sticks to sour sticks - into glucose (blood sugar). The key factor is the rate of that conversion. The slower the body metabolizes the glucose (low glycemic), the more stable the blood sugar level, resulting in a less ravenous appetite and consistent, extended energy – which is what we want. The faster the conversion (high glycemic), the more unstable the blood sugar becomes which triggers a spike and crash of energy, stimulates cravings, feeds our fat cells and fuels a rush of insulin – all of which we don't want. In addition, the sugar also goes to the same part of our brain's reward system, releasing pleasure sensors such as endorphins and dopamine.

THE CONTROLLED EATER VS. THE COMPULSIVE EATER

The same dynamic applies here: the "controlled" eater can take one or two cookies and stop. Even though they're consuming refined carbs and experience that temporary reward pleasure, the intensity and sensitivity is not as acute as with a compulsive eater. As well, the instability of their blood sugar isn't as precipitous. The highs aren't as high, and the lows aren't as low. A perplexing yet profound way to encapsulate it is: If you can say "no," then you can say "yes." If you can't say "no," then you can't say "yes." Or alternatively: one is too many because then 100 is not enough. Try digesting those ideas.

And the act of compulsive overeating can elicit the same responses even without the abundance of refined carbs. It was many the night that I binged on a bucket of fried chicken and super-sized fries. The comfort, escape and emotional anesthetic--not to mention the sheer indulgence--can generate a compulsive reaction and reward mechanism in a person who may have such a disposition.

Perhaps one could suggest that food is the most abused drug in the world. It's legal, widely available, and quite possibly the focus of more direct and subliminal advertising than any other product in history. And we have to eat!

I want to reiterate at this point that by no means am I representing myself as a physician, medical scholar, or scientific expert. I'm merely sharing with you my understanding based on my extensive research and learning, as well as observations drawn from the more than fifteen years of exposure and coaching I've had with thousands of overweight and obese people – and my own experience of struggling with, and recovering from morbid obesity. There's an abundance of credible information available online. Here's a link to just one example from the National Institutes of Health on a study titled: Evidence for sugar addiction: Behavioral and neurochemical effects of intermittent, excessive sugar intake. https://www.ncbi.nlm.nih.gov/pmc/articles/PMC2235907/.

I highly encourage everyone to do your own thorough exploration and drawn your own conclusions.

GOOD CARBS VS. BAD CARBS – AND ROBUST CALORIES VS. EMPTY CALORIES

To begin formulating a path toward recovery, we need to tease out the distinction between good carbs and bad carbs, and robust calories vs. empty calories. As well, it's crucial to recognize that there are two halves to most addictions, the physical compulsion and the mental obsession. In order to achieve long-term success, it's vital to address both.

Carbohydrates are found primarily, but not exclusively in grains, vegetables and fruit. When we consume the whole food in its most natural form, such as whole oats – commonly called old-fashioned oats, or a whole orange, our body is breaking down the food more slowly because it's beginning the digestive process in a less refined and more whole form. The glucose conversion rate is mitigated by the fiber in the food as well as the intrinsic fact that the body is doing the refining, and therefore breaking down the food at a more moderate pace.

However, if we consume orange juice, or a product made from oat flour, the glycemic rate is elevated because the food is beginning the digestive process in a much more refined and concentrated state. We're refining the orange by extracting the juice (which houses the sugar) and processing the oat grain by grinding it into flour *before* it even enters out mouth.

THE WHOLE GRAIN VS. WHOLE GRAIN BREAD VS. WHITE BREAD

ANATOMY OF A GRAIN

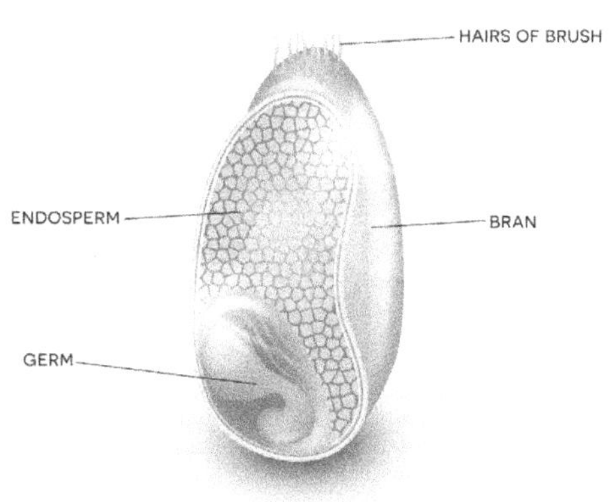

What's in a grain, anyway? A list of the most common grains includes: wheat, oats, barley, spelt, and rye. There are three primary components to each: the bran, the germ, and the endosperm. The bran and the germ contain the lion's share of the nutrients and fiber, and the endosperm is the fluffy, white substance.

White bread is processed by first removing the bran and the germ, leaving the nutrient-deficient endosperm to be milled into flour. Whole-grain bread is more nutrient rich because it's milled into flour with its three original parts. Don't be fooled by "enriched" or "fortified" white bread, which means "manufactured" nutrients have been added back into the white flour. It's not same as your body absorbing the naturally occurring nutrients from the whole grain.

So, is whole-grain bread (the most popular being whole wheat) healthier than white bread? For sure. But – and this is a big but – *it is still a refined food*. Why? Because any time a grain is ground into flour, that -- by definition -- is refining it by pulverizing it into tiny particles, and therefore accelerates the glucose conversion.

This is highly relevant for the compulsive eater because we are much more sensitive to any accelerant which can create a greater instability in our blood sugar, which in turn stimulates cravings. My experience is that there are varying levels of tolerance even among people who exhibit compulsive eating tendencies or history. Some can tolerate moderate to minimal amounts of more refined carbs on occasion, while others can't.

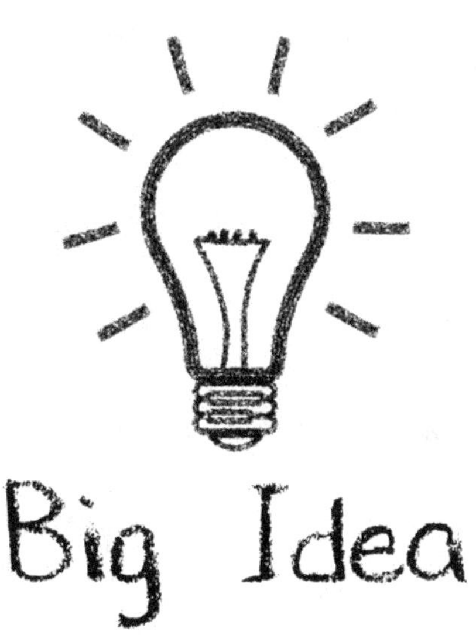

That's why the Soveya Food Plan suggests to prioritize whole foods and to try and minimize all refined carbs, whether they are whole grain or not. And that's certainly beneficial for everyone, whether you self-identify as a compulsive eater or not.

For example, hot cereals such as old-fashioned oatmeal in the morning instead of bagels or donuts and cooked whole grains or starches for dinner like brown rice, potatoes, or quinoa instead of pasta or noodles. Rice cakes (made from puffed rice instead of rice flour) are even a better alternative for a sandwich than most breads. There's a litany of luscious choices to make that can provide us with the nutrients we need from grains without having to fall back on the refined carbs.

In addition, all of these products – think bread, pasta, cake and most breakfast cereals – are often loaded with sweeteners and preservatives in addition to being produced from flour. The golden rule is: the fewer the ingredients and/or the added sweeteners, the more ideal the choice.

And that holds true even for no-calorie sweeteners – whether they are artificial or "natural." Because they still stimulate your sweet tooth, perpetuate cravings, and can actually increase your appetite.

NOT ALL CALORIES ARE CREATED EQUAL

The next step of our puzzle is to gain the skill of discerning between robust and empty calories. I'll give you an extreme example, but it will clearly illustrate the picture.

Let's say that an optimal daily caloric consumption for both Simon and Larry is 2,000 calories. Simon gets his calories from three meals consisting of lean proteins, grains, vegetables and fruit. Larry, on the other hand, fasts all day and then eats a 2,000-calorie massive cotton-candy stick at night. You don't have to be a nutritionist to figure out that their bodies will react very differently, even though they are consuming the exact same number of calories.

Why? Because the cotton candy is the classic case of empty calories. It's void of any nutritive value. It has no protein, healthy carbs, fat, vitamins, minerals, or water. Zero for six. A big goose egg – and not nearly as nutritious.

So what happens to those 2,000 calories of sugar – otherwise known as refined carbs? They give Larry a very short burst of energy by spiking his blood sugar, which then quickly crashes and stimulates cravings and an insulin rush – and ends up mainly just feeding his fat cells.

In stark contrast, Simon's healthy cells are sufficiently

nourished from the nutrient-rich calories he ingested, giving him extended energy, satiation, and optimum health. Since this is his ideal caloric intake, there are scant excess calories and no refined carbs, resulting in conscientious and consistent weight loss if needed. He is simultaneously nourishing his healthy cells and starving his unwanted fat cells. Now that's hitting the real daily double.

As we can now understand, this demonstration is also extremely important for the compulsive eater, because the more excess and/or empty calories we consume, the more we prolong this vicious cycle of spiking and crashing our blood sugar with all its deleterious effects. And the body's detoxification can be a highly uncomfortable but nevertheless extremely important process. The more we minimize the refined carbs, the more we maximize our health and decrease our physical dependency.

DISAPPOINTING OR DEVASTATING?

But unfortunately, that's just half of it. It'd be so much easier if we could just go through a few days of agonizing physiological withdrawal and come out on the other side with a complete freedom from food obsession.

However, the emotional attachment we have developed with our "security blanket" of compulsive eating is just as concrete a connection and irrational affection as Linus and his. If you don't know what I'm talking about, ask someone over forty.

I postulate that the DNA of a craving is twofold: how much we enjoy it and how upset we are by not having it: 1) the emotional currency we invest in that immediate physical gratification delivered by the double-fudge brownie; 2) the perception of the profound deprivation and loss if we don't have it. *"I just can't live without my ____"* fill in the blank.

We're distraught and devastated when we don't get our "fix." We literally panic. Not just because our body craves it, but also because we have a demonstrable fear of restriction when it comes to our eating. We pity the fool who tries to get in our way or dares to deprive us of what we so desperately "need."

And this is the crucial self-maturation process we must work through in order to completely and finally free ourselves from food obsession and achieve long-term success.

When I tell someone I haven't gone on a rollercoaster for seventeen years, they don't give it a second thought. When I tell them I haven't had a piece of chocolate cake in seventeen years, their eyes bug out, their jaw hits the floor and they stare at me as if I just walked off the set of *The Twilight Zone*. "Such control, such self-discipline," is the customary feedback I receive. Allow me to burst your bubble.

I'm going to call upon each of you now to summon your unconditional honesty to answer the following question: Is there really a difference between the two?

Let's say twenty-year-old Sarah and her six-year old niece Miriam really love rollercoasters. They make a plan for just the two of them to have a special day together at the amusement park next week, highlighted by a ride on the craziest, loopiest rollercoaster there. Miriam is waiting with bated breath. She's counting down the days, then the hours until the time finally arrives to get in the car and leave. They arrive at the parking lot, run right through the turnstile, right past the bumper cars, the laser tag and the arcade until at last they reach the rollercoaster. There's just one problem – it's surrounded with yellow tape and signs proclaiming, "closed for repairs." Sarah's response at that moment? "Oh, that's such a shame." And Miriam? She's devastated and breaks into an inconsolable tantrum.

Why? Why is it that even though the enjoyment level relative to the both of them is equal, they have such disparate reactions when that pleasure is taken away?

The answer is that Sarah is not emotionally invested in those two minutes and forty-five seconds of excitement. Sure, it'd be fun to do, but it's not such a big deal if she doesn't have that experience. It's disappointing but not distressing.

Miriam, on the other hand, is completely invested in that immediate gratification. It's the most important thing to her at that moment. Nothing else matters. She's emotionally all in, as well she should be. She's six years old. That's completely normal and understandable. That's why she's shattered.

And therein lies the formula for emotional maturity: the ability to process a feeling, not necessarily be overwhelmed and overrun by it. It's a growth process that we have all undergone in so many aspects of our lives, knowingly or unknowingly, intentionally or organically. We all have those muscles and possess that skill set. Now, we have to apply it to our relationship with food: to refine the way we think and feel about eating, changing our head and our heart, to be unconditionally honest with ourselves.

The piece of chocolate cake is nothing more – and nothing less – than a two-minute, forty-five-second rollercoaster ride for our taste buds. That's all it is, and all it will ever be. When that connection is made, we experience a palpable palatable pleasure. Without a doubt. But again, for just those two minutes and forty-five seconds.

There's always going to be delicious chocolate cake around somewhere. And I don't advocate taking a scalpel and scraping away our taste buds, even though that would probably be a more effect weight-loss surgery than a bariatric bypass.

So, if we can't change the ingredients of the cake, and we aren't going to change our taste buds and the subsequent reaction when those two meet, then what can we change? The answer is: we can change how important that reaction is to us, how emotionally invested we are in that immediate gratification.

It's okay not to go on the rollercoaster. Really, it's okay.

Especially for those of us who always come off the ride feeling nauseous, sick, and incapacitated for the rest of the day. That temporary thrill is never worth the cost. There are other rides that are fun but don't pack the same baggage. Bumper cars instead of the rollercoaster.

And It's okay not to have that piece of chocolate cake. Really. It's okay. Especially for those of us who perpetually suffer the regret, remorse, discomfort, and distention of yet another binge. It's never, ever worth it. I promise you that you'll not just survive, you'll thrive.

Just like there's an amusement park loaded with "healthy" rides, there's a supermarket full of healthy foods that will stimulate our taste buds and support our wellbeing. We don't have to 'sacrifice' that palatable pleasure in order to experience that immediate gratification. We just have to be willing to access it from a different source – bananas instead of a banana split.

We don't need to be intuitively creative in the kitchen, or a trained gourmet chef to create simple yet delicious dishes that promote our health and wellness – insert here a shameless plug for our Soveya Cookbook. But we do have to be willing to step outside of our comfort zone to try new foods and resensitize our tastes to the naturally occurring flavors

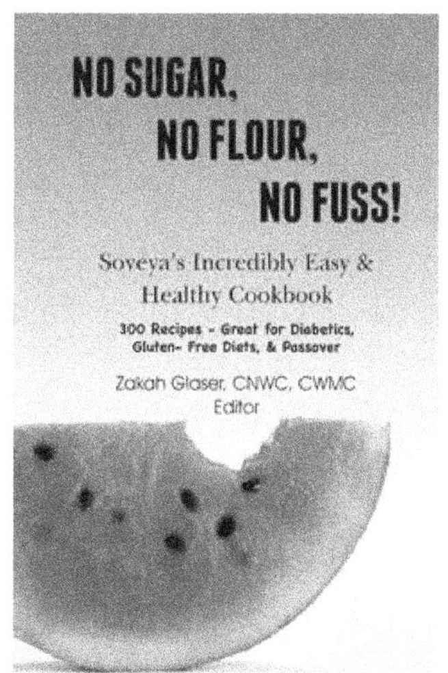

that inherently exist in less refined and processed options. Truthfully, is there anything wrong with that? Didn't our palatable palate expand from when we were five? Who says it has to stop now?

Concretizing this realization and committing to this process was the root of my transformation. I wasn't accessing some new-found willpower, self-control, or discipline. I was willing to be unconditionally honest with myself and my immature relationship with food. It didn't mean I was a bad person. It did mean that I had to be willing to change my attitude toward food and attachment with binge eating – changing my head and my heart.

And that's the process of self-maturation in our relationship with food and freeing ourselves from the mental obsession. And we can do that only within the boundaries of a well-defined food plan. Because we need to keep those wires of spontaneity disconnected on a daily basis.

PROACTIVE ABSTINENCE VS. PASSIVE ABSTENTION

There's still one huge question that begs to be answered in our ongoing comparison. Here's the scenario:

Michael is a recovering alcoholic who has been maintaining his sobriety for many months. Gabe is a former compulsive overeater who has just reached a healthy goal weight after losing more than 100 pounds.

"Michael," you ask, "are you sober today from your compulsive drinking?"

"Yes," he says with a huge smile.

"What does that mean, exactly?" you add as a follow-up question.

"Very simple," he says. "I just didn't put my hand on a drink today."

Now you turn to Gabe. "Have you abstained from compulsive eating today?"

He says, "Yes," with the same wide grin.

And then you continue in the same manner, "What does that mean, exactly?"

If Gabe's answer is the same as Michael's, "I just didn't put my hand on food today," that'd be a very inappropriate answer. Why? Because Gabe – like all of us – *needs to eat.* Starvation is not a recipe for health.

Even though Michael and Gabe are standing shoulder-to-shoulder at the finish line of recovery, they arrived via very different paths. For all other behaviors – whether it's alcohol, gambling, or drugs, the definition of daily success is very simple: You either drank or didn't drink; gambled or didn't gambled; used or didn't use. It's a distinct demarcation.

By no means am I implying that it is easy, effortless or in any way belittling such a huge accomplishment. I believe that any addict who is active in clean recovery is a role model for all of us to emulate in regard to changing behaviors and lifestyles that can seem overwhelming and unattainable.

All I'm doing is identifying that the definition of sobriety is very clear-cut. It's called passive abstention – they avoided engaging in that substance or behavior. They didn't cross their bottom line.

We can't say that about eating.

Which begs the question, what was Gabe's path to the finish line? How did he end up standing next to Michael at the end of a successful day if he had to engage in that behavior that he was trying to avoid in the first place? Quite a conundrum.

The answer lies in examining from what was Michael really refraining? When he said he didn't pick up a drink, what that really means is that he didn't pick up his will, his spontaneity, and impulsivity with alcohol. He may have had a thousand reasons to rationalize the need for a drink, but he didn't validate them with an action. As tempting, inviting, and intoxicating as it felt, Michael chose not to act on that feeling. No matter how excruciating it was, he decided not to pick up.

For even though he would have been powerless over that second drink, he didn't have to pick up the first drink.

Addiction is often summarized as self-will run riot. But you don't have to let the horse out of the barn, no matter how hard it's bucking.

So how does a compulsive eater not pick up his will if he has to pick up food? It's called staying inside the blue box. The Soveya Food Plan is a color-coated tapestry of food groups, goals, and guidelines. But sitting on top is the blue box – delineating how many meals, and/or snacks for the day, and from which groups to choose for each. It's a personalized GPS, exquisitely navigating a person through their nourishment from morning till night.

Gabe certainly has the autonomy to select which food from any particular group he wants for that meal, e.g. cheese, yogurt, or eggs for his breakfast protein that morning. But if he sticks precisely to the prescribed quantities listed for each choice and adheres to the specific groups and schedule of meals, at the end of the day, he has successfully picked up food but not his compulsion.

He may have woken up late and wanted to skip breakfast, but he made the time anyway. He may have been in the mood for a mid-morning muffin, but he didn't indulge. His co-workers may have brought in pizza and cake for a surprise office party, but he stuck with his lunch that he brought from home. He may have been ravenous for more chicken at dinner because it was so delicious, but he stuck to his portion. He may have been stressed at night from the bills and craving the mint-chocolate chip ice cream in the freezer, but he stayed away.

At the end of the night, Gabe put his head on his pillow having remained within the firm borders of the blue box – no matter what temptations, feelings, or impulses may have beaten away at him. He stood shoulder-to-shoulder with Michael at the finish line of a successful day, but via the path of proactive abstinence instead of passive abstention.

He felt his feelings but didn't eat over them. He didn't allow his impulsive thoughts about food, either by commission or omission, to manifest into action. He was well aware that his compulsive eating would have been triggered yet again if he reconnected those wires of spontaneity, if he gave himself permission to act on that momentary desire, no matter how subtle or serious the digression.

He fully understood that he would have been powerless over that second bite. But he was also fully aware that he didn't have to take that first bite – no matter what.

And when he woke up the next morning, Gabe was showered with the three reinforcements of success even before he got out of bed. Firstly, he didn't regret following his food plan and refraining from his temptations. He didn't say to himself, "On second thought, I wish I had actually thrown away my lunch and joined the pizza party or polished off the whole pint of ice cream last night."

Secondly, he felt good about himself, cherishing the sweet taste of integrity and accomplishment that comes from having stuck with a goal regardless of how challenging it seemed. As well, he felt physically good, not bloated and distended from sleeping off another binge.

And thirdly, he looked back with keen 20/20 hindsight and acknowledged that it wasn't as hard as he feared it would be – the perception of the degree of difficulty is so often greater than the actual degree of difficulty. These three reinforcements serve as the foundation upon which to build another successful day – the building blocks of the blue box. For Gabe truly integrated and experienced the reality that: *Nothing tastes as good as feeling good feels.*

THE PRIORITY PYRAMID

Now we see why boundaries are so essential in changing our relationship with food – and why this is so relevant, whether you self-identify as a compulsive eater or not. This paradigm is a productive protocol for change for anyone looking to improve their eating habits.

Because at the end of the day, it's not a weight problem or a nutrition problem – it's a behavior problem with adverse nutritional and body-weight consequences. Here we go again, distinguishing between the problem and the consequence. Eli, you sound like a broken record. Guilty as charged. I have a compulsive tendency to follow the following adage: *The main thing is to keep the main thing the main thing.*

You could certainly argue that there are three priorities

addressed when following the Soveya Food Plan: 1) weight loss; 2) sound, consistent nutritional choices; 3) abstaining from compulsive eating behaviors. Which one are we going to crown on top of the priority pyramid?

Well, if our perspective is to merely treat this as another diet, then we might place weight loss as the highest goal. But is that going to really affect a long-term solution? Probably not. Because then we can rationalize skipping meals or skimming from the plan here or there to "jump start" our weight loss. And what have we done in the process? We have renewed our license to make arbitrary decisions around food – again, either by commission or omission, which could then easily reopen the barn door and awaken the sleeping bronco of compulsivity.

Same as if our main objective is to "eat healthy." That will also allow us to justify another fruit here or there, or some more nuts on occasion, or a few extra pieces of sweet potato just because they taste so good. After all, we can say to ourselves, they're not refined carbs. What's the big deal?

Trust me, it's a big deal.

What if you happened upon our friend Michael at a pool party a few months later and you see him grabbing a wine cooler from the ice chest. You run over to him and with a friendly yet concerned look and ask, "Michael, what are you doing?"

"Hey, it's just one wine cooler," he says. "It's not such

a big deal, just 'fruit juice with an attitude.' It's not the bottles of scotch and vodka I used to drink all the time. I'll be fine."

Technically, he's right. Fruit juice with an attitude means it's has just a splash of alcohol mixed in. But you don't need to be a professional addiction counselor to know he's fooling himself and about to dive in very deep and hot water. Why? Because that one wine cooler could easily lead to the second and third, and then the scotch and vodka.

What did Michael really pick up when he grabbed the wine cooler? He picked up his self-will and reconnected the wires in his brain of impulsivity with drinking – regardless of what the actual soldering agent was.

Therefore, the core function of our food plan is not to effect weight loss or consistent nutritional choices. The primary purpose of the plan is to create a method and medium to achieve proactive abstinence. If we make that our crowning priority, then we'll realize real and lasting behavioral change – and, by the way, will reap the wonderful and crucial benefits of long-term weight loss and healthy eating. That's not just hitting the daily double – it's cashing in on a true trifecta.

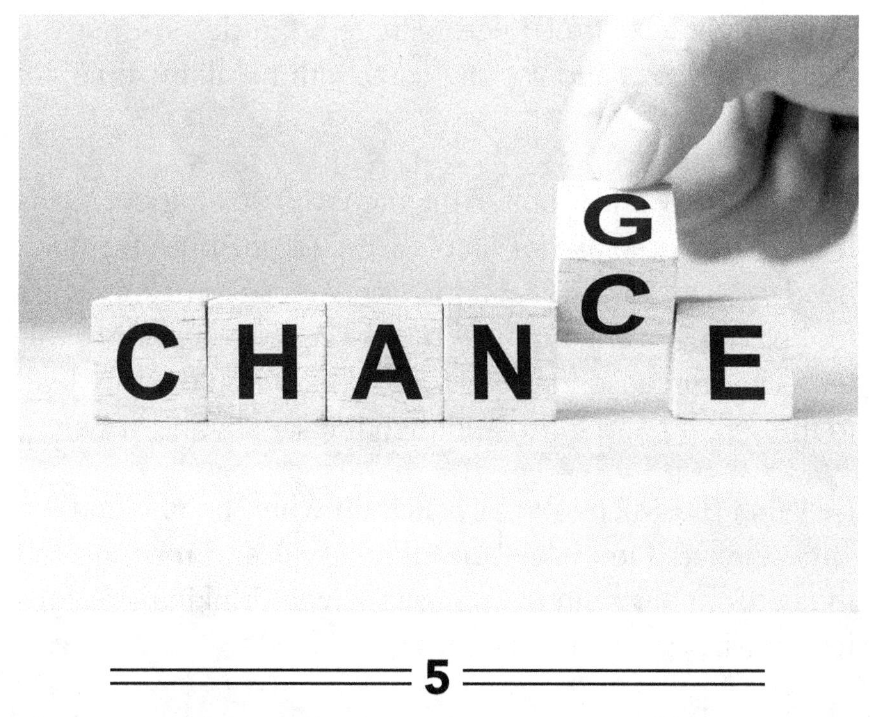

5

KEY ONE: C.H.A.N.G.E.

NOTHING CHANGES IF NOTHING CHANGES.

Seems simple and cryptic at the same time. Actually, it's one of the most profound ideas I'm going to share with you.

Chances are that you - along with millions of others around the world – have probably tried a few – or a few dozen – diet programs and/or products on the market. Think of the one common theme that unites them all.

Here's a small sample of real advertisements. I'm not making this up.

"New herbal extract melts body fat while you sleep!"

"Anti-obesity pill cuts out need for exercise or healthy eating!"

"Special supplement burns as many calories as a four-hour workout!"

"Diet meds scientifically proven to block fat and eliminate cravings!"

"The cookie diet!"

"The pizza diet!"

"The dessert with breakfast diet!"

"The ice cream cleanse!"

And the list goes on and on. So again, what's the common theme underlying all these promotions? The answer is: We don't have to do any work to get the results we want. We don't have to give up our favorite foods or change our lifestyle in order to change our body size.

Think about that for a second. Is there anything else in life where someone would have the audacity to offer us a genuine achievement without any investment of effort or accountability?

What if there was:

"The 90-minute law-school degree!"

"Ten days to becoming a board-certified cardiologist!"

"Earn your commercial pilot's license through new video game!"

The humor is eclipsed only by the absurdity.

So why is the multi-billion-dollar diet and weight-loss industry replete with these programs? Because the human psyche has a palpable fear of change. Our body's set point is inertia. We crave comfort and loathe exertion. That's the natural resistance that exists in all of us. It doesn't make us bad people, just part of the human race.

Ask anyone the following question, "What's the opposite of pleasure?" What will most likely be their reflexive answer? "Pain. Pain is the opposite of pleasure."

Close, but no cigar.

Pain is not the opposite of pleasure. Pain is actually a major ingredient in attaining pleasure. No pain, no gain.

When I speak of pain, I'm not referring to the agony of a toothache or broken leg. Pain in this context refers to the discomfort involved in exerting the necessary effort to achieve a genuine and meaningful goal.

For in fact the greatest aspirations and achievements in life require the greatest effort. Let's take raising kids for example. Ask a parent, "What's your greatest pleasure?" They'll say, "My kids."

Ask them, "What's your greatest pain?" They'll say, "My kids."

That's not a contradiction. The greatest effort (hopefully) they invest in life is in their children, which generates (hopefully) their greatest joy and satisfaction.

I can attest to that first hand, as my wife and I are blessed with the wonderful pleasure of rearing our five wonderful kids. I'm not going out on a limb when I say, "It ain't easy," – even though they are really easy kids.

Having picked up the "hobby" of distance running a few years ago, I experience this same phenomenon during the course of a race. Completing 26.2 miles doesn't come easy to me. But having endured and crossed the finish line at events such as the New York City Marathon, the Marine Corps Marathon – and especially the unbelievably hilly Jerusalem Marathon – were simultaneously the most arduous and exhilarating feats of my life.

No pain, no gain.

If that's the case, then what is the opposite of pleasure? Glad you asked.

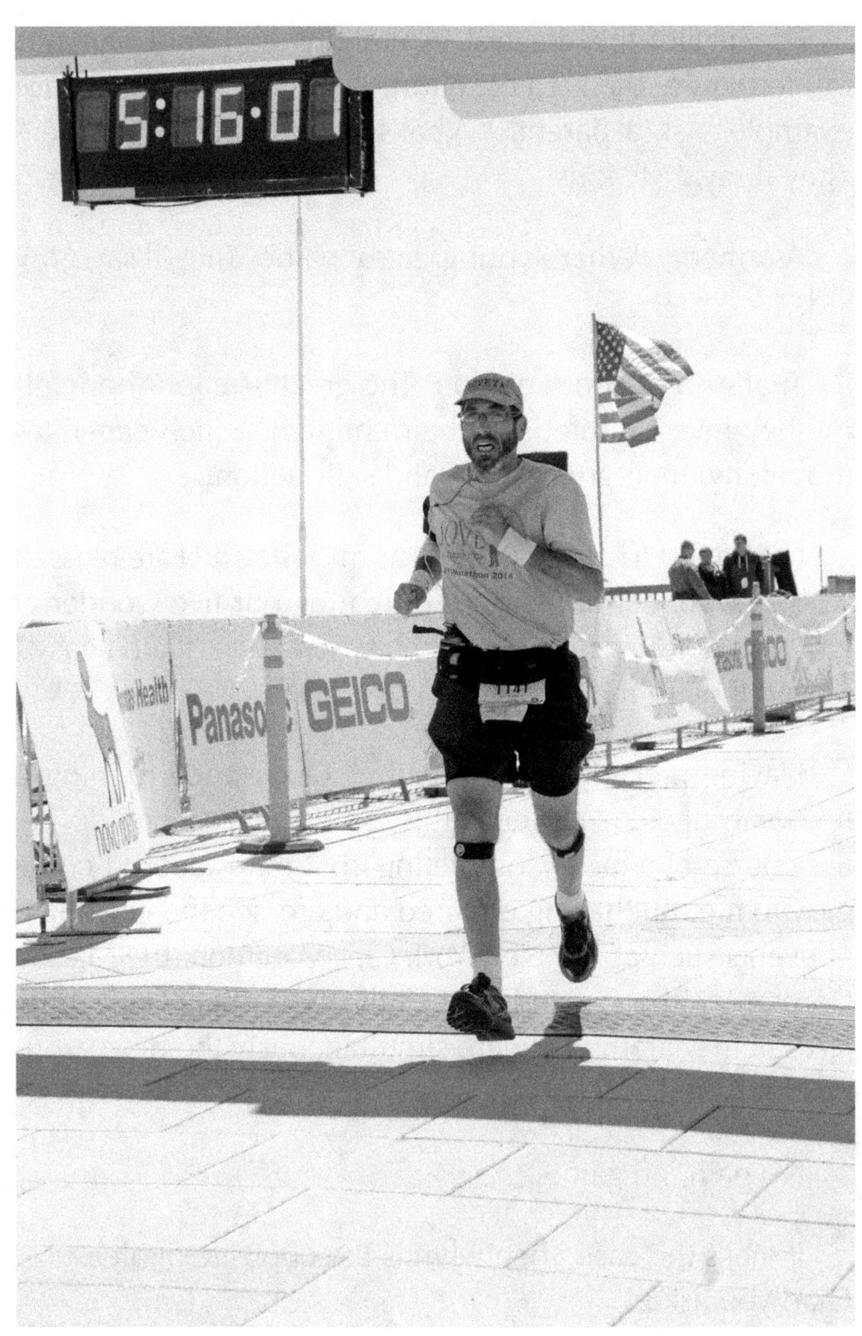

New Jersey Marathon

The opposite of pleasure is comfort – otherwise described as "lack of effort."

Now, there's nothing wrong with sleeping in a comfortable bed, with a cozy pillow and a lush blanket. But hopefully, that's not our goal in life. And we certainly don't want to go out of our way to make things difficult in our lives just to prove a point. Trust me, we'll encounter enough challenges along the way without having to manufacture any.

Our aim is to be willing to exert any effort required to pursue reasonable and responsible goals which are in our best interest to achieve.

And the daily objective for all of us is to push through our particular blocks and venture outside our comfort zone. It's called waking up in the morning, going to work, feeding the kids, or studying for the test even though we don't *feel* like it. We acknowledge our feelings but move past them, attempting to put the next foot forward and do the next right thing. Progress instead of paralysis.

It's called maturation and responsibility. These are not earth-shattering concepts, but rather the basic building blocks of human achievement. To the extent of the resistance is the growth. To the extent of the effort is the reward.

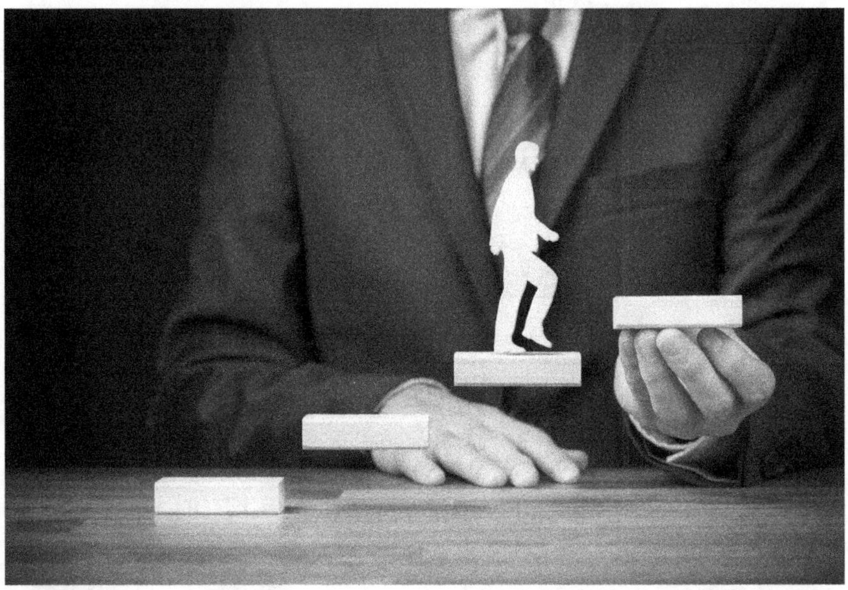

For example, if you begin strength training for the first time, you don't necessarily start with 25-pound weights, because that could overwhelm you and you wouldn't even get off the ground. The level of resistance has to be suitable for each individual in order to initiate movement. Therefore, you might start with the 5-pound barbells for the first couple weeks.

But if after a year you're still curling the 5-pound weights, chances are your muscles wouldn't grow at all. You need to appropriately add resistance in order to effect change.

It's called progressing through the life cycle of human development; moving on from kindergarten to elementary and high school – college, profession, relationships, marriage and family. We would never condone or encourage ourselves or our children to be perpetual third- graders.

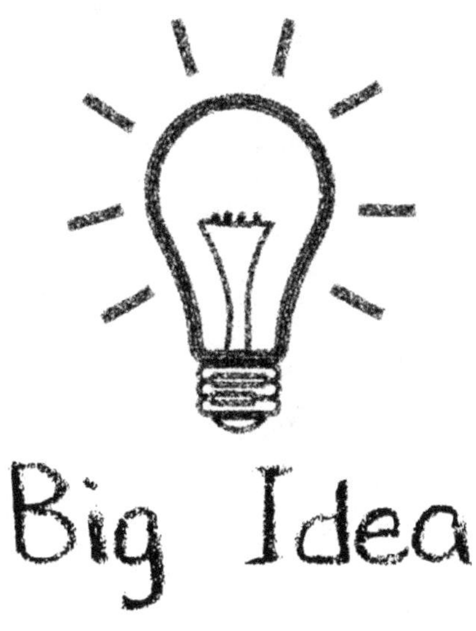

Change stimulates growth. Complacency causes stagnation.

That's why C.H.A.N.G.E. is the first of the Seven Soveya Keys to unlock your blocks and propel you toward success. It's the master key, the ring that connects all the others and perpetuates the progress in transforming your relationship with food.

C.H.A.N.G.E. stands for:

Courage
Humility
Accountability
Necessity
Gratitude
Enthusiasm

These are what I call the six essential attitudes of change. You don't necessarily have to master these attitudes. But you must be willing to embrace them, because stepping outside of your comfort zone requires the willingness to change. And if you want to permanently change your body size, you have to change your attitude and actions when it comes to eating. There's simply no other way to achieve lifelong success.

The sooner you stop searching for the magic pill or secret shortcut, the quicker you'll gain traction on the road toward recovery. Are you ready to stop spinning your wheels?

C – **C**OURAGE

Let's start with the letter **C**. I could have easily gone with **C**ommitment, **C**larity, or **C**onsistency – which are in fact vital components in our tool belt of success of which I often speak.

But I chose **C**ourage, because I firmly believe that this is the necessary first step toward change. For, as we see, change means to confront and conquer our comfort zone. One small step of progress often requires a giant leap of faith in ourselves.

To even contemplate living without the companionship, comfort, or emotional crutch of food can be highly disconcerting. Perhaps it's simultaneously been our best friend and worst enemy for much of our lives. Entertaining the thought of abandoning fast food, convenience eating, or impulsive indulgence is harrowing.

Picture the scene. Dave was born with a birth defect in his leg, requiring him to use a cane in order to walk. When he was thirty-five, doctors developed a ground-breaking procedure that could cure Dave of his limp. He gladly underwent the surgery. The orthopedist visited Dave in the post op, informing him of the smashing success of the operation.

What's his first reaction – to hop out of bed and begin tap dancing? Of course not. Dave must endure exhausting physical therapy to learn to put weight on his leg for the first time in his life without use of a crutch. Dave needs to summon up the courage to take those first, few painful steps. He's gingerly walking down the hallway of the hospital screaming at the physical therapist to give him his cane. His discomfort is genuine. A crutch is all he's known his whole life.

The PT is going to give him encouragement, support, direction, and advice. But he's *not* going to give Dave the cane.

Why does Dave voluntarily engage in this discomfort? Because it's temporary, and the necessary cost of change. Each day brings a little more progress, and a little less pain. Before long, he's walking down the street with a clean and energetic gait, indistinguishable from anyone else. Courage was the accelerant that fueled his drive, blazing a path toward persistency and perseverance.

Dave is a hero and an everyman at the same time. For we all have the innate courage to summon the necessary fortitude to encounter and eclipse our personal stumbling blocks.

Especially when it comes to food, because unlike Dave, the crutch of food is more perception than reality. If we're in the throes of emotional anxiety and for whatever reason don't have access to our nerve-numbing nosh, what will honestly and objectively be missing from our lives the next morning? Nothing, other than the regret, remorse, and extra pounds resulting from another binge.

We need the courage to walk through, and work through our fears. Because in our unhealthy relationship with food, F.E.A.R. stands for ***F***alse ***E***vidence ***A***ppearing ***R***eal (see upcoming chapter for an in-depth discussion of this key). We *feel* that we can't survive without our comfort foods, or that healthy eating is too hard, burdensome, and depriving.

Even though those feelings appear real to us, they are in fact false. Accessing the internal courage to admit that and to broach the boundaries of our comfort zone is the first step toward real and lasting change.

H – *H*UMILITY

Do you want to know the biggest meal I had to digest while beginning my road to recovery? A huge slice of humble pie – without the whipped cream, of course.

One of the most prodigious pitfalls preventing many of us from incorporating real and lasting changes in our eating habits is a lack of humility. And I don't mean self-centered arrogance.

Okay, now that you're really confused, let me explain. The initial independence we all achieve in the course of our lives is managing our own eating. Parents are thrilled when their baby can hold the bottle on their own, or the first time they can successfully maneuver the banana into their mouth instead of stuffing it up their nose.

These are moments of celebration and marked accomplishments. The inauguration of our sense of self is directly associated with our ability to self-nourish.

The two grow hand-in-hand as we grow through life. It's natural, normal, and necessary. We know what tastes, textures, and flavors we favor – what's sweet and stimulating, and what's sour and unsavory.

It's an intimate and ongoing experience. And even if we've reached a point where we realize a need to change – whether to lose weight, avoid foods that don't agree with us, or address health concerns – we still look at it through the lens of "I know what *works* for me." We harbor our habits very close to our vest.

Therefore, the humility we need to engender in order to facilitate thorough and lasting change is not the abandonment of egotistical arrogance, but rather, the willingness to be teachable at whatever age, stage, and station of life we're in – to welcome and embrace change and learn new behaviors.

We're not self-absorbed, supercilious snobs. We might have fuller faces as a result of our overeating, but we're not necessarily bigheaded. The humility I'm talking about is not an antidote for haughtiness.

It's the combination to unlock the block of self-sabotage.

When it comes to a complete commitment to comprehensive change, we often get in our own way. We trip ourselves up because deep down we think we know better – based more on duration than denial.

After all, we've been feeding ourselves since we were weaned. It's an ingrained trait that's part and parcel of our personality. It's disconcerting, and even disorienting, to recognize that our relationship with food is a liability in our lives – that in order to reach the goals we desperately desire, we need to develop the willingness to wipe the slate clean, to dive down as deep as necessary to unearth any and all harmful habits that have hampered our ability to institute a healthy relationship with food.

Engaging unconditional honesty in confronting detrimental attitudes, obsessions, and fixations with food is crucial in allowing the underpinnings of change to take hold. And humility is the foundation upon which honesty can root.

A – **A**CCOUNTABILITY

Parents and teachers. Coaches and consultants. A sponsor or a spouse. In addition to supplying love and support, education, and guidance, a common seed they all plant in us that enables our potential to sprout forth is accountability. Overtly or covertly. With words or with deeds. Silently, or even by their mere presence.

When we have someone to whom we're accountable, we will exert effort and energy to a much greater degree than we will if we are left to our own devices. It's the rare individual who can generate sufficient internal combustion to power their way toward achieving their life's goals. And even they need standards of success against which to measure themselves.

One of the magnificent manifestations of mankind is the realization that we don't all live on our own isolated islands. We depend on each other to survive and to thrive. It's not a weakness. It's a reality.

The attitude of accountability stands on the broad shoulders of humility – for, once we are wholeheartedly receptive to suggestions and direction, we can then adopt those changes in our daily eating behaviors and be comfortable and committed to the scrutiny of success. We're willing to be vulnerable enough to expose our mistakes and share our victories, not for the purpose of critical condemnation or false flattery, but for sincere support, encouragement, and correction.

It's a common denominator found in all of us, even world-class athletes. We'll work harder and push ourselves more if someone is standing over us. Being pulled past our comfort zone is a much smaller step than if we have to leap it on our own, even though it's really the same distance.

It's so easy and accessible now. A text or a tweet. A

phone call or email. Engaging an accountability partner is a paramount priority for change.

And that's the difference between a coach and a cheerleader. Both will applaud and congratulate when the player succeeds. But when the player stumbles, the cheerleader sits on their hands and says nothing, while the coach gives direction and advice. That's his role and responsibility. In fact, the player is paying him big bucks to do just that, because the player understands that only through accountability will he be able to meet his goals and push past his comfort zone to a level he may never have reached on his own.

In my work with clients, I call it the three A's for effective coaching: Advocacy, Accountability, and Action. Besides providing a clear action plan of change and advocating to prioritize their personal needs in the face of their other taxing professional and family demands, I hold my clients accountable to their own aspirations. Not just with weekly weigh-ins, but objectively examining their attitudes and activities to see if they are in concert or in conflict with their goals. To be constructive and caring, empowering and empathetic, positive and practical.

And I'm constantly reminding them that I'm doing it for their sake, not mine. I'm here to help them in any and every way I can. They don't pay me to tell them what I think they *want* to hear; they pay me to tell them what I think they *need* to hear. I'd be negligent if I did anything less.

If we don't have someone to whom we answer, it'd be so much easier to succumb to the momentary craving instead of calling upon the courage, clarity, and commitment to work through that feeling, regardless of how uncomfortable it might be at that instant.

I can attest to that first hand. For years I was the reigning monarch of rationalization when it came to giving in to my obsession for self-indulgence. And the reams of regret I wrote out the next morning didn't translate into change until I had the willingness to be held accountable by someone else. I finally threw away my broken glasses of self-perception and was willing to look at my eating behavior through the lenses of another person, who shared his clarity, wisdom, and vision. Only with that prescription was I able to successfully navigate my way toward real and lasting change. I've been seeing 20-20 ever since.

N – ***N***ECESSITY

Luxury or necessity--you make the choice. It's only a matter of life and death. No big deal.

One of the most influential people in my life shared this brilliant idea with me: The real definition of wisdom is not the ability to tell the difference between what's important and what's not important (although that is certainly a helpful skill) – it's the ability to distinguish between what's important and what's *more* important.

I'm going to go out on a limb and venture to say that 99% of the people reading this book are not independently wealthy, living lives of constant pedicures and manicures, three-hour leisurely lunches and monthly vacations. Our lives are filled with taxing demands on our energy, time and patience, professionally and personally. And multiply that by ten if you have a family with kids.

Simply put, we have a lot of important things to do each day. That's a given. But what's the *most* important responsibility we have? Managing our own health. Period – or "full stop" as they say on the other side of the Atlantic.

I call it the significance scale. We can determine the importance of something with two criteria: 1) How much of it is in our control to make happen; 2) What's the consequence if it doesn't get done.

Let's use the example of being a teacher or a parent. Those are pretty darn important positions in life. They have huge impacts on their students and children – to educate, support, encourage, and provide effective role models. Really big stuff.

But at the end of the day, the kids are still independent people who are going to make their own decisions. Therefore, the level of control a teacher or parent has is significant, but certainly not absolute. And the consequence of being a dysfunctional teacher or absentee parent is also astronomical. But we've seen the incredible resilience of children to overcome these setbacks and thrive in life.

So, I would certainly score a parent with a 9.5 on a scale from one to 10, and teachers are also pretty high up there.

Apply the same standard to any number of roles and responsibilities we have in life, and we'll see where they fall on our significance scale. We do it all the time while dividing our never-ending to-do list into luxuries and necessities. A luxury is something nice to accomplish, but if it doesn't happen, it's not such a big deal. The necessities are the things that we prioritize because something meaningful will be missing if we don't get it done.

Which brings us to eating – or more specifically, changing our relationship with food. How often do so many of us relegate our daily nourishment to the lowest rung of our priority ladder, commonly skipping breakfast, eating on the run, grabbing a little something here or there and then inevitably making up for it by stuffing ourselves later in the day, or endlessly noshing at night. Been there and done that. Guilty as charged.

A common cause of obesity is under-nourishing during the day and over-nourishing at night. Breakfast really is one of the three most important meals, for no other reason that it sets your metabolism to a high point soon after waking up, enabling you to have sustained energy and most efficiently burn calories throughout the day.

"I'll pick something up if I can," is a common and seemingly harmless refrain, but nevertheless still a massive misprioritization of our time. Why?

Because our self-care through proper nourishment is *the most* important responsibility we have to fulfill every day. It trumps everything else. Everything.

Yes, even more important than taking care of our children. Wow, that seems like a pretty provocative statement. Let me explain.

When you're getting ready to take off on a flight, the attendants review the safety instructions. "In the event of a loss of cabin pressure, oxygen masks will fall from the ceiling. If traveling with small children, put your mask on first."

Why isn't that a classic case of child neglect? Because if you're encumbered, you can't properly care for your children.

Changing your relationship with food – being willing to do whatever is necessary to heal your body from being overweight or obese and to break lifelong habits – has to be your primary priority day in and day out. An attitude of "necessity" is essential for success.

Your food plan is the constant, and your schedule is the variable—not the other way around. Meaning that your breakfast, lunch, and dinner are the three most important appointments of your day. Without exception.

There's no greater gift you can give your children than a healthy parent. And I guarantee you that 99.99% of the time, you'll be able to do both. You'll have the time, energy, and focus to take care of all the other important necessities on your hectic schedule – including child care – while still prioritizing your self-nourishment as number one.

In fact, if we're open and honest about it, you'll be much more capable of fulfilling your other roles because you won't be weighed down, physically, mentally, and emotionally with your food obsession. You'll be healthier, freer, and more engaged.

And to bring it all together, self-nourishment scores a 10 out of 10 on the significance scale. Because it's the only thing in this world that we solely do for ourselves. We are the final arbiter of what goes in our mouths. We make that choice. No one else.

G-d forbid we should ever have to be in a situation where we need to outsource our nourishment to someone else – where we're so incapacitated that we're incapable of feeding ourselves or lose the ability to swallow that we require the nutrients to be tubed directly into our stomach.

Which brings us to the second criterion: What's the consequence if it doesn't get done – if we don't improve our relationship with food and continue to prolong the behaviors that have got us to this point? I'll answer that with the following true story.

Sammy, a good friend of mine, has a buddy name Jack. Jack was a really overweight guy who suffered a massive heart attack. Following emergency bypass surgery, the doctor came into his room and said quite bluntly, "If you don't want your wife to be a widow, and your children to be orphans, you must change your lifestyle right away."

Well, Jack certainly got the point, and for a few months he was really make great choices and prioritizing his health. But then one evening, Sammy ran into Jack at the buffet table at a wedding reception, pounding away at the fried chicken wings, sucking the meat and skin off the bones like a skilled artisan. Plate after plate kept on disappearing. Sammy just stood there in abject silence, until he mustered up the fortitude to ask the obvious question.

"Jack, what are you doing?"

"These wings are great, Sammy, especially the bbq."

He asked again, "Jack, what are you doing?"

"These are delicious, man, the best wings I've had in a long time."

He asked again, this time with a little more incredulous tone, "Jack, WHAT ARE YOU DOING?"

"What do you mean, 'what am I doing,'" Jack responded as he licked the sauce from his fingers. "What does it look like? I'm eating wings."

"No," said Sammy. "You're not eating chicken wings. You're spitting in the face of your children by telling them that a chicken wing is more important to you then they are."

And with that, Sammy walked away.

Luxury or necessity, you make the choice. It's only a matter of life and death. No big deal.

G – ***G***RATITUDE

E – ***E***NTHUSIASM

Adopting an attitude of gratitude and lighting a fire of enthusiasm are essential for sustained success and round out the key of C.H.A.N.G.E.

Think of all the common terminology of dieting. "I'm being strict. I'm being strong. I'm sacrificing. I'm depriving myself." It's all about struggle and conflict. We voluntarily put ourselves in jail in order to hold ourselves back from those foods we really want but are being "good" now so we can lose weight. We do it begrudgingly. It's a necessary evil.

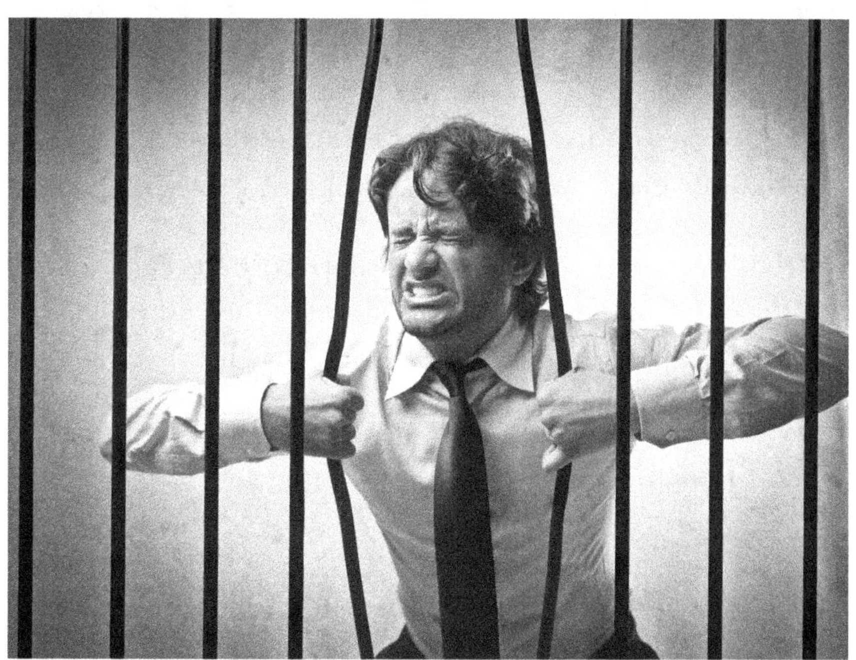

We resent having to change – having to put limits on ourselves. We're bitter about having to eat vegetables, even if they aren't bitter herbs.

We look forward to the "cheat" when we can sneak in that cupcake when no one's looking. But in the end, we're just fooling and cheating ourselves.

This self-destructive attitude is a sure-fire formula for failure. So why is it that we so often engage in this self-sabotage? Because we're coming at it from the entirely wrong perspective. We're trying to lose weight as quickly and as effortlessly as possible.

We're not interested in genuine change. We want the results without the effort. We want the rewards without the investments. We just want a diet that works – but we don't want to have to do the work.

In my dictionary, D.I.E.T. is a four-letter word, literally and figuratively. It usually ends up spelling: **D**id **I** **E**at **T**hat?

That's why we perennially end up frustrated and suffering from diet fatigue. It's not that we're insincere. It's that too often our expectations and goals are misplaced.

An attitude of gratitude and an energy of enthusiasm is the ultimate power-steering fluid that helps us turn the wheel in the right direction.

Let's revisit the story of Dave, who had the major

operation to fix the birth defect in his leg. He knew full well what he was getting into. The whole procedure – the complicated surgery and grueling rehab--were meticulously laid out before him. Despite all the effort and discomfort that were to commence, he said yes anyway. Enthusiastically. He was enormously grateful for the opportunity to change, even with all that it entailed.

Why? Because he knew that was a better alternative than remaining in his current condition. And he accepted that this was the only way to achieve the result he so desperately dreamed of. His physical therapist came up with a motto for Dave to repeat daily. Every morning he showed up for therapy, he was asked, "What are you doing today, Dave?" And he said with a smile, "Whatever it takes."

We don't need invasive surgery or painstaking physical rehabilitation to achieve our goals. What does "whatever it takes" mean for us? To stick to our food plan no matter what. To feel our feelings instead of feeding them. To be comfortable being temporarily uncomfortable. To feel the freedom to say "no" instead of feeling burdened to say "no."

We can have two prescription schedules presented to us to address our diabetes, high blood pressure, high cholesterol, and hypertension. A litany old Latin-sounding meds like Metformin, Clonidine, Lipitor, and Furosemide – not to mention the onerous CPAP machine for sleep apnea. Or a food plan prescribing a robust and clearly defined regimen of fruits, vegetables, proteins, and grains.

Herein lies one of the great open "secrets" about weight loss and obesity. It's in our hands to change. More often than not, we can greatly reduce – if not completely eliminate -- the need for these drugs by just changing our eating habits, developing a healthy relationship with food, and maintaining an appropriate body size. Is there anything to be more grateful for than that?

We should enthusiastically embrace the effort, not be burdened by the bitterness.

When asked every morning, "What are you going to do today to stick to your food plan?" Everyone smile and repeat after me, "WHATEVER IT TAKES!"

"It really is amazing when you follow the food plan how the cravings go away. The chocolate demons have departed! I also love the mantra 'whatever it takes.' That has really kept me going."

– Amy, Chicago, Illinois

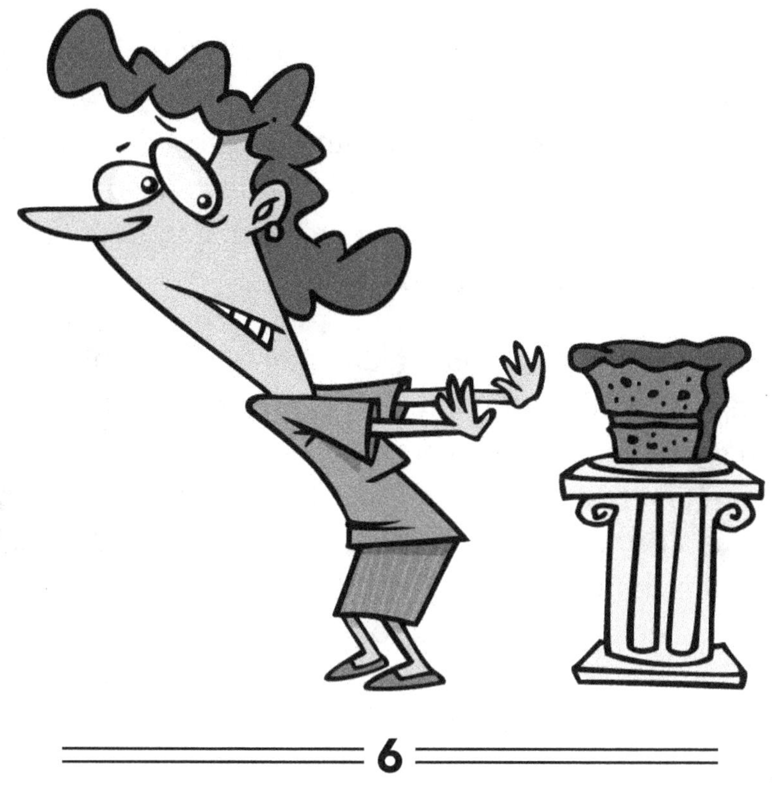

6

KEY TWO: H.A.L.T.

Just because we're hungry doesn't mean we need to eat.

The next key we must secure after firmly grabbing the master ring of C.H.A.N.G.E. is to become a skilled and keen diagnostician. What's really going on inside us when we feel the desire to eat? Does it necessarily mean our body is lacking nutrients? Often, it doesn't.

The four basic triggers for all mankind that generate a

feeling for food are represented in the word HALT – standing for: Hungry, Angry, Lonely, Tired. These are the four universal situations in life that either create a craving, and/or which we associate with eating. And we need to follow the intrinsic definition of the word and stop (halt) before inexorably reacting with food.

Don't hit the panic button and flail for food on that first feeling. Hydrate and contemplate – drink and think. We need to stop, take a deep breath – and preferably a glass of water – and reach out for reason. That's certainly the more reasonable and responsible response than stuffing our face upon that initial instinct. And that's exactly the personal development we're looking to cultivate and concretize as we transform our relationship with food – to react reasonably instead of irrationally. What a concept!

Let's break down these four categories.

***H* - *H*UNGRY**

Going an extended period of time without eating causes the glucose levels in our cells to drop, resulting in a lack of energy and stimulating a signal in the body to refuel. This is the quintessential indicator of "healthy" hunger.

Just like the censor in our car's gas tank illuminates the warning light on our dashboard when it gets below a certain threshold, so too the intricate systems in our body monitor the energy supply in our cells and generate a physiological sensation when it's time to replenish. At that point, we need to restock with a robust supply of the six essential nutrients necessary to survive and to thrive – and I don't mean a handful of supplements.

This is what's called "healthy" hunger, because it's the body's legitimate need for nutrition. And therefore we need to respond accordingly by nourishing ourselves with the ideal quality and quantity of food. That's why the timing of our food plan is so imperative – the T. in the Q.Q.T. By adhering to the scheduling parameters of our plan, we will avoid the extended chasms between meals and not put ourselves in this compromising situation.

If we earnestly and honestly commit to this process, the incidents where we find ourselves - through no fault of our own - legitimately delayed from our next meal by some extraordinary circumstance will be very few and far between. And even then, in those rare situations, we'll be able to deal with those uncomfortable moments by concretizing our commitment that "vulnerability doesn't have to equate inevitability" – just because we're compromised doesn't mean we have to cave in.

Our glycogen reserves will power us through until our next meal. Will it be pleasant? Not necessarily. But, assuming we're not diabetic, hypoglycemic, or possessing any other acute medical condition, we'll survive. And if we are in one of those categories, then our food plan should be responsibly customized to account for those scenarios – giving further credence that cookie-cutter, one-size-fits-all diets don't have your best interests in mind, and in the end don't help you get to that one size into which you really want to fit.

But again, if you ensure that your self-care through proper nourishment is the ultimate accomplishment of your day, these episodes should occur seldom at most. Keep your fingerprints off the panic button.

But as we learned previously, there's a flip side as well to legitimate hunger. It's called appetite. Once we embark on the fueling process, the fun can easily override the function, causing us to overeat. Just like Miriam who was engrossed in playing with her friends and didn't want to end that fun time, the same dynamic is in play with us when we are consumed with a delicious consumption and don't want to stop just because we reached our objective limit.

Let's say that six ounces of protein is the appropriate amount for Hank. If he goes out to dinner and is served a 10-ounce prime rib, what's his normal reaction upon finishing the forkful that completed the sixth ounce? He wants to keep on going. Just like Miriam, Hank's in the middle of an enjoyable experience and naturally wants to continue. There's nothing pathologically wrong with him for having that feeling. It's perfectly normal, but nevertheless not necessarily the choice he should make – even if it's a choice cut.

It's uncomfortable to push the plate away at that moment, staring longingly at those final four ounces of his new "friend." What's going to fuel his clarity and constitution to commit to such a counterintuitive action? It's called the key of HALT. He's going to stop before he goes forward with the next forkful, reminding himself that the feelings he's having about food from this point onward are not his body's need for nourishment – even though physiologically there's absolutely no difference in the sensation from one moment to the next.

Better yet, Hank will use the key of HALT as a pre-emptive shield before the steak is even served. He'll make it a point to create an awareness and mindfulness to anticipate an upcoming conflict, knowing full well that he'll soon be in the throes of a palatable pleasure and that his instincts will create a momentum for more, but that he still has the capacity to hover over the brakes and step down when arriving at the six-ounce stop sign. It won't automatically make those few moments any less uncomfortable. But it will give him the focus and resolve to do the right thing, even if it isn't immediately rewarding.

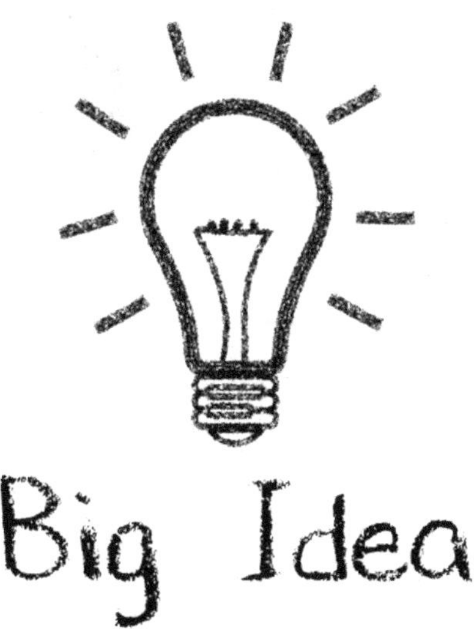

The car is not going to stop on its own. But just because he's hungry doesn't mean he needs to lay the pedal to the metal. And upon giving himself those few minutes to digest the food and "step away from the plate," the sensation of satiation will start slowing down the momentum and take the edge off his drive for more.

And the more Hank habituates himself with this behavior, the more he'll actually be teaching his body the skill of satiety, rendering those immediate physical desires for more less intense and less frequent. Now, that's real satisfaction.

A - **A**NGRY

Anger or anxiety, stress or sadness, disappointment or displeasure – these are common expressions of emotional discomfort and turmoil. What's an innate inclination for many of us at this point – one that has also been ingrained in our collective psyche since time immemorial? To soothe ourselves with something sweet. Or sour. Or spicy. Or to stuff down our feelings by stuffing our face. Eating as a means to alleviate stress is a product of both nature and nurture practiced the world over.

Comfort food. It's an industry within an industry. Alluring and appealing. Inviting and intoxicating. We energetically embrace it during our greatest vulnerability and scorn it contemptuously during our contrite occasions of clarity--the ultimate bittersweet relationship.

Now before we get too ahead of ourselves, the key of HALT is neither the time nor the template to teach you how to break the bonds of emotional eating. We will address that in depth in a later chapter. Not to worry.

What we are doing at this point is fine-tuning our

diagnostic skills of self-assessment when it comes to cravings and desires – to develop an awareness and understanding that lifelong habits and ingrained tendencies don't necessarily equate healthy behavior. The focus of this key is to build the skills of intellectual anticipation and behavioral response to an impending susceptibility, so our actions don't have to replay the same regretful reaction.

Vulnerability doesn't have to equate inevitability. Just because we feel like eating doesn't mean we HAVE to eat. The chauffeur driving the car of emotional consolation may pull up to our door delivering a dozen donuts of delightful distraction, but we can still choose not to get in if we honestly diagnose our feelings and focus on the foreseeable destination of dejection and despair to which we will inevitably be driven.

Take a pass and pass the water. Hydrate and contemplate. It's just not worth the trip.

***L* – *L*ONELY**

Food is fuel, not a friend.

There are times in life where we all may find ourselves lonely for companionship or bored for something to do and wouldn't you know it, the next thing we know our head is in the fridge looking for the next exciting fifteen-minute activity. How'd that happen?

We gravitate to the kitchen almost by osmosis – magnetically and mindlessly driven on a mission to eat that has absolutely nothing to do with our body's need for food. For years, I traced tracks in my house from the living room to the kitchen that were so well worn you would think they were part of the original design of the wood floor.

The bell in my belly would ring and off I went like a Pavlovian dog, dutifully determined to dig out my next dish. Downtime meant dinner time – even if I already had packed away a full supper. Only with the key of HALT was I able to stop and begin the process of processing my feelings instead of feeling compelled to have to act on them.

We can learn to enjoy our own company, and better enjoy the company of others, if we're not confounded and consumed with thoughts of consuming. And, quite frankly, we'll feel more comfortable in our own skin if it's not bursting from our bloated bodies.

That's the senseless, self-destructive pattern that many of us perpetuate: We isolate because of our perceived inferiority fueled largely by our large size, which creates a lack of friendship or comfort to commingle with others, which triggers a sensation for food to fill the void of loneliness.

Rinse and repeat. Rinse and repeat. That's one shower we never walk out of feeling cleansed and refreshed, only soiled and sullen. But we can put a HALT to that practice by anticipating those first sensations and put in place a pre-emptive plan to respond to those feelings for food without having to feed ourselves. Choose three alternative activities to access at those moments – such as taking a walk, calling a friend, or writing in your journal.

Step outside of yourself just for a few minutes to regain your clarity. And you'll see an amazing thing – that these three categories of triggers are just what they represent – ALT – an alternative feeling toward food – not an objective need to eat.

T – *T*IRED

One of the most significant skills I gained in the transformation of my relationship with food was the permissibility and prominence of sufficient self-care. I used to erroneously equate it with self-indulgence. If I felt like eating because I was tired – using food to fight the fatigue – it must mean that my body needed it at that time. Wrong diagnosis.

I needed rest, not raisin bran.

Following a well-regimented food plan, day after day, helped me rework the wires in my brain that boundaries weren't binding, but building – even if it went against my immediate inclinations. And that in turn helped me to put boundaries around other areas of my life. Like late nights.

I started to cut them out.

Even though I felt like staying up late – often just for the sake of that anticipated midnight snack --I learned to do a radical thing: I went to sleep. Wow, what a revelation.

Actually, for me it was. I would abuse my body by either working too hard, playing too hard, and most of all, eating too hard.

Over these past seventeen years, I have learned to prioritize my rest, whether that means trying to go to sleep at a more reasonable time, or sometimes taking a twenty-minute power nap during the day – without feeling guilty. I'm no longer perpetually propping myself up with caffeine hits from diet sodas, but rather, hydrate myself with water, which supplies extended energy by helping to support steady blood sugar.

And here's another "insider secret"--I'm way more productive now than ever before. Not being weighed down, literally and figuratively, I'm much better equipped to maximize the sixty minutes of each hour.

Because the more we push ourselves beyond a reasonable limit, the more fatigued we get, and the more we have the tendency to turn toward food for a quick kick.

And that brings us to the last point which ties this key together: We should try to avoid these triggers as much as possible, aiming to not get too hungry, angry, lonely, or tired.

Granted, some of these circumstances are out of our control. But you'd be surprised how many are in our hands to regulate. Because we're not merely undergoing a change in our weight, we're undertaking a change in ourselves and in our relationship with food – which positively impacts so many other areas of our life.

And, therefore we can abide by the adage that just because we're hungry doesn't mean we need to eat.

"I'd like to share with you an anecdote that occurred on the way home from an overseas trip. It was a night flight, thus I had already eaten my third meal of the day according to my food plan. The flight was supposed to leave at 9 p.m. We boarded half an hour late, and then had another delay of an hour or so until take off. Later, I just couldn't fall asleep for a couple of hours.

I felt so bored and restless. At first, I was feeling a bit sorry for myself – I have seven hours of sitting on this flight, and I can't even eat anything, and nothing else with which to distract myself. Then I remembered six years previously, coming home on a similar night flight and bingeing non-stop. I ate whatever was in sight: packets, buns, sweets, airline food. I remember it so clearly, the way I was stuffing my mouth nonstop. Needless to say, the aftereffects were horrible.

And remembering that, I resolved to be grateful. Grateful for the fact that I could actually sit for seven solid hours, with no distractions, and not even think about bingeing. Grateful that the following morning – I would wake up and eat a regular breakfast, without feeling drugged up and ill from overeating."

- Rachel, London, England

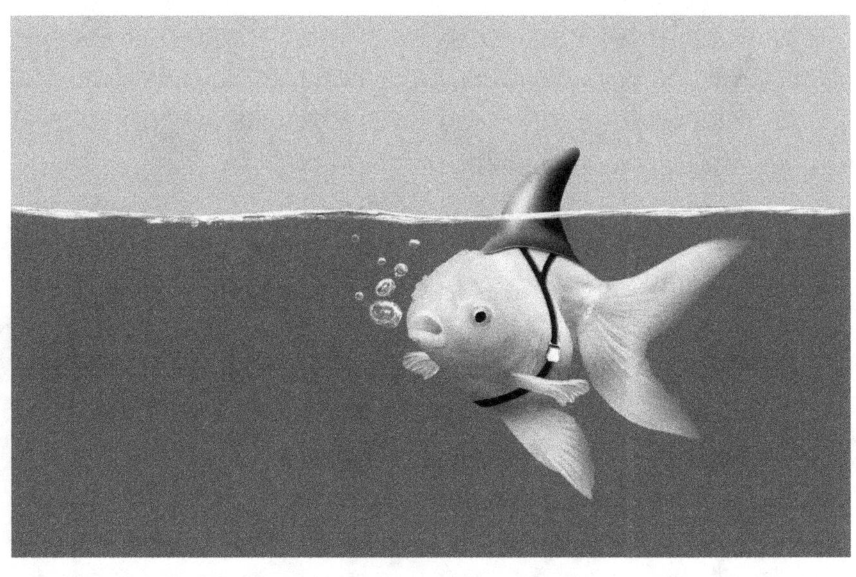

7

KEY THREE: F.E.A.R.

***F**ALSE* ***E**VIDENCE* ***A**PPEARING* ***R**EAL*

Deprived. Restricted. Starving. Sacrificing. These are some of the palpable fears that paralyze so many people from making meaningful changes in their eating habits, and the funny thing is, they don't even realize it.

One of the most pertinent questions I ask all my clients during their initial evaluation is "What are you afraid of? What do fear is holding you back from enacting a complete and comprehensive overhaul in your relationship with food?"

The question catches them off guard. They often look at me quizzically, not associating the emotion of fear with their history of frequent failed attempts at maintaining a weight loss or even sticking to a basic diet plan.

"I don't want to be hungry but I'm not afraid of it."

"I'm not afraid of feeling deprived. I just don't like restricting myself."

Guess again.

Fear-based inaction is one of the primary spike strips that flatten our tires and incapacitate us from making real progress down the road of recovery. And that's why learning to confront and conquer our fears is critical for our success and ranks as one of the Seven Soveya Keys to unlock your blocks.

The reason many people don't quite comprehend the question at first is because they understandably interpret it as referring to the primal fear of someone sneaking up behind them in a dark alley. The chocolate cake may rob us of our integrity and health, but it won't steal our wallet and jewelry.

The fear to which I'm alluding is the deep and disorienting distress of having to break habits and eclipse emotions that we inwardly project to be part of the very fiber of our being.

Throwing away that security blanket of spontaneity that has "shielded" us for so long is demonstrably disconcerting. It's been our singular point of reference for comfort and support since we began perceiving food as our core source for consolation. We literally feel we have no other place to turn.

Whether eating is our pacifier, protector, or primary port of unbridled pleasure, ridding ourselves of these behaviors is a Himalayan climb which we feel woefully inadequate to crest.

That's the evidence that appears real to us – painstakingly and paralyzingly so. But that's because we're looking at it through our faulty prescription. Our lenses are colored, coated by our innate insecurities around food, reflecting a rose-colored glow on the inside to what is objectively a sight of sickness and sorrow that lies right beyond our nose. And that's the ironic sadness of it all; we deliriously desire the binge foods as seen through our skewed vision but can't smell the accompanying foul stench of the aftereffects that will inevitably engulf us each and every time.

It's time to whip those glasses off your face, toss them on the ground, and stomp them into little shards. Because the evidence that appears real to you is not. It's false. It's F.E.A.R. – false evidence appearing real.

You can absolutely attain satiety and security while sticking to a sensible and satisfying food plan. Spontaneity is not a sanctuary. Impulsivity doesn't provide immunity to life's challenges. Unrestrained quantities don't result in uninhibited pleasure, just a momentary thrill followed by extended anguish.

We feel that we can't survive without our comfort foods, or that healthy eating is too hard, burdensome, and depriving. Summoning the courage to walk past these fears begins with looking at them for what they truly are – false flames of a fiery doorway through which we dread to pass. We're paralyzed by our perceptions instead of fueled by facts.

It's like the toddler who refuses to go to bed without a parent in his room. Eventually, the mother decides it's time for young Johnny to learn to fall asleep on his own. She tucks him in, kisses him good night, and walks out of the room.

He begins to wail. Five minutes, ten minutes, maybe even a half hour. Upon each sob, the mother feels like a knife is plunging through her gut, but she steadfastly sticks to her resolve and doesn't walk in. Eventually, he tires out and falls asleep.

The same scenario plays itself out over the next few nights, but each time it takes less and less time for Johnny to fall asleep, until the evening soon arrives when little Johnny goes right to sleep with a smile on his face.

What transpired? What changed? The mother helped Johnny walk through his fears. There was no bogeyman under the bed, or monster in the closet lurking in Johnny's vivid imagination, waiting to jump out when the coast was clear.

By walking over the threshold of his bedroom door, his mother wasn't abandoning him forever, but merely helping Johnny develop the confidence and awareness that his environment was completely safe and secure despite his initial perceptions to the contrary.

It was an uncomfortable yet invaluable experience -- much like most of life's maturation process.

Fast forward a few years. Johnny is getting ready to get on the school bus for the first time in his life. He has more than a little trepidation, maybe even a tear or two in his eyes. He fears a nasty bus driver or unfriendly kids preparing to make his life miserable. His mother comforts him and lovingly wipes away his tears but doesn't validate his fears. She doesn't say, "You're right, Johnny; the bus driver is really mean, the kids are all brats, and therefore you shouldn't get on the bus."

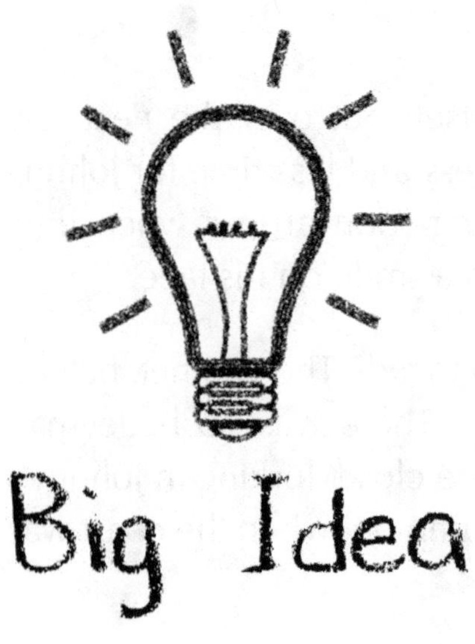

She tenderly and encouragingly helps him alight the steps, thereby facilitating another instrumental life lesson – that the evidence rooted in subjective perceptions that appears real to us isn't always so. In fact, it's often false. Learning to walk through – and work through -- our fears is an emboldening and elevating experience, even with the requisite discomfort.

Let's examine these fears as they relate specifically to food:

HUNGER

"I can't go around all day being hungry. I'll go out of my mind." Or, as they say in my neck of the woods, "I feel like I'm gonna plotz!"

Those could be reasonable and realistic associations based on past experience with reckless crash dieting. However, like we learned in the previous key of H.A.L.T., if we have a robust and responsible eating plan, then any alternative sensations of hunger are not necessarily indications of our body's need for food.

The first flicker of hunger triggers an alarm, creating a convoluted conclusion that we can't withstand the next few minutes without satisfying that sensation. We must, therefore, abandon our previous priorities and grab that first thing available to appease the abdominal uproar. We fear that if we don't act with alacrity, it will escalate to overwhelming proportions.

Sounds like heightened hyperbole? Not at all.

That's the evidence that appears real to us – that we will suffer from unbearable discomfort if we don't immediately satiate our hunger. We'll be distracted and incapacitated from normal functioning if we don't eat something right away.

Not true. We will survive. With the Soveya key ring firmly in our grasp, what's going to be our first reaction from this point forward? Hydrate and contemplate. Drink and think. Down some water and process the feeling. Wait those five uncomfortable minutes for the sensation to simmer down and the water to saturate inside. Work it through; don't let it work you over.

Recognize that you ate a full meal just a little while ago and your next meal is coming soon. Another meal is always coming. You'll be left alone only if you abandon the food plan. And that's never a pleasant island upon which to be stuck.

DEPRIVATION

Another manifestation of the six-year-old syndrome is the dread of deprivation. When we see other people enjoying a "forbidden fruit," it often instantaneously generates a wide-eyed wanting that didn't exist merely two minutes prior.

Picture the scene: Robert is working hard at his desk, focused intently on the task at hand and feeling no hunger. Then his co-worker brings in a steaming hot pizza pie, the smell of which is wafting through the office creating a magnetism no less powerful than The Pied Piper's melody.

Bob's attention is turned immediately to the contents of the flat cardboard box; his stomach begins to rumble, and his mind starts to race. Those reactions – in and of themselves – are not abnormal, but his emotional interpretation is definitely detrimental.

"I can't believe they get to eat the pizza but not me. That's so unfair. I have to stick to my crummy diet while they can dig in. If I don't eat something now, I'll be distracted and won't be able to work for the rest of the day."

He was fine five minutes before. Nothing physiologically changed in his nutritional needs other than his assessment that he is now depriving himself of a few indulgent moments. If Bob's co-worker took a different route to his cubicle and therefore Bob was never aware of the pizza party, he would have maintained his productivity none the wiser.

His judgment that he is now severely compromised from maximizing the rest of his day is in error. Bob has allowed his erroneous emotional evaluation to gain enough traction that it has derailed his objective decision-making ability.

He is now paralyzed by fear instead of fueled by facts, resulting in joining the gathering for a slice or sulking to the vending machine for some bittersweet solace. Either way, Bob is no better off now than he was before.

On the contrary, by feeding his irrationality he continues to sanction his spontaneity under the guise of a necessary reaction to a temporary discomfort, which perpetuates the problem instead of seeding the solution.

This same paradigm is manifest in other unsettling life situations, such as a tactile need for comfort and security or diverting our thoughts and feelings from loneliness and boredom. We have habituated ourselves to believe that the only way we can cope with these conditions is with the antidote of food. We are convinced that there is no other option. That evidence appears painstakingly real in our eyes.

But in reality, it's painfully false. We have to access the attitude of courage to propel us past the threshold of our comfort zone and be willing to experience these circumstances without the crutch of cupcakes. Only by putting blinders on our skewed vision will we be able to move forward and walk through our fears. In our mind's eye it seems like the edge of a cliff, when in actuality it's the first few steps toward real freedom.

"I'm getting used to the meal plan and don't feel deprived. I feel healthier and have more energy. I used to feel food had power over me; now I have the power. I control the food instead of it controlling me. Even my kids are eating healthier, eating more fruits and brown rice because they see what I'm doing. It's amazing."

- Andrea, Santiago, Chile

LEAVING
COMFORT ZONE

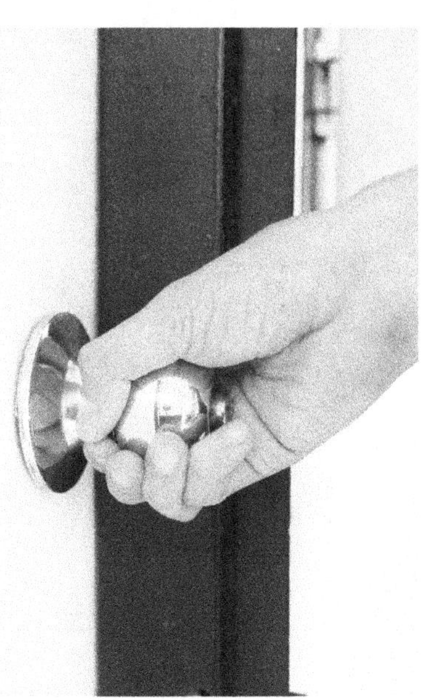

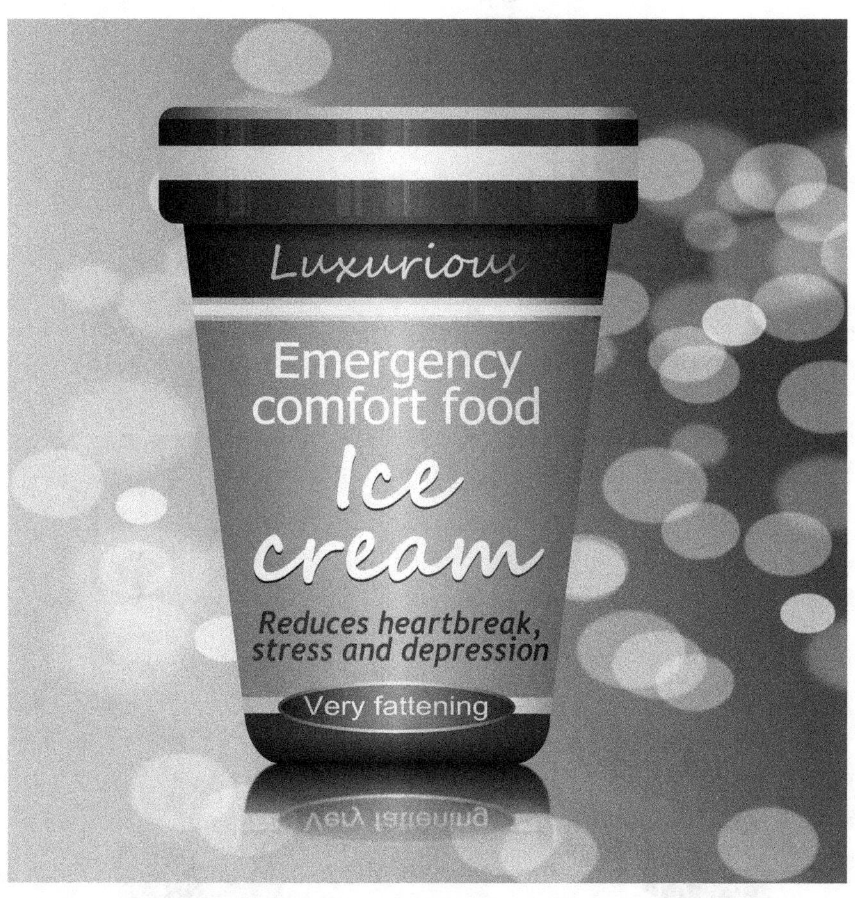

8

KEY FOUR: FACE YOUR STUFF, DON'T STUFF YOUR FACE

(Breaking the Bonds of Emotional Eating)

Charlie is walking down the street and starts to feel an irritation under the bottom of his left foot. He soon realizes that a pebble must have gotten in his shoe. That's no fun. It's definitely uncomfortable.

How is he going to manage the problem? He's got four options.

Four, you ask? Only one is most likely to come to mind.

Option A. He can head straight to the emergency room of the nearest hospital and demand that they amputate his left foot. That would certainly eliminate the irritation under his heel. But it's probably safe to say he won't opt for this option – perhaps a touch too radical of a response.

Option B. While he's in the hospital, he can plead with them for a huge needle full of Novocain to completely numb his foot. Would that eliminate the irritation? Yes. Is it less extreme than cutting off his extremity? For sure.

So, would he go this route? Undoubtedly not. Why? One reason is that if he became habituated to this response it may end up damaging the nerves in his foot. And a more compelling reason not to choose the anesthesia is that he has a much simpler solution – which brings us to . . .

Option C. Charlie would find the closest place to stop on the street, lean on something to take off his shoe and shake out the pebble. At this point you may be asking, "Eli why did it take you 234 words to state the obvious?"

And additionally, once we presented the last and most

straightforward scenario, what could possibly be a fourth choice? Glad you asked.

Option D. Let's say, for sake of discussion, that there is no convenient place suitable for Charlie to stop and take off his shoe. What's he going to do then? Being of sound mind and body buttresses him from electing either of the first two irrational alternatives, which leads him to the only remaining possibility-- he'll continue down the road, bearing the discomfort until he reaches his destination.

The pebble is a pain, but it's not incapacitating. He'll deal with it until he can deal with it – he's not going to debilitate himself to deal with a discomfort, nor anesthetize himself to alleviate an annoyance.

FRITOS INSTEAD OF FEELINGS

You might not have given it much thought, but food is probably the most universally accessed anesthetic. We eat to sedate our stress, distract our discomfort, placate our pain, and even numb our everyday nuisances. Our emotional eating is not intended to solve our problems. That much we know. We're using comfort foods to temporarily take our minds off of our issues.

We're using food as a sweet and soothing sedative. It's not *like* a drug. It *IS* a drug – the most abused drug in the world. It's legal, easily available and more proactively promoted than any other licit or illicit contraband around.

We're rash to rationalize our self-diagnoses and secure in the fact that we can always write our own prescription. We can literally diagnose, prescribe, and order our meds all while remaining prone on our personal examining table – giving a whole new meaning to the term "couch potato" -- that's, of course, if we add fries to the pizza delivery.

So how do we break this vicious cycle? How can we come clean and learn to live life on life's terms without the ever-present dependency on a cheese Danish? I'm not exaggerating when I say that I've had more than one client that could not leave their house without the security of a Snickers bar in their pocketbook – tear wrapper in case of emergency and bite down.

Our first step is to unconditionally acknowledge that not only does comfort eating fail to solve our problem, it always creates a second problem – in the short term and long term. The short-term cost is in the form of exacerbating the physical and mental impact of our weight gain and obesity, which certainly bears prolonged consequences as well. The additional long-term price is that the perpetuation of this behavior stifles us from developing healthy and productive coping mechanisms for life's challenges.

The prize in the Cracker-Jack box doesn't contain the solution for our difficulties. There are no answers in the Almond Joy, and polishing off a pint of Rocky Road doesn't ease our path – remaining true to its name.

What do all of these things do? They make us feel good

for the moment, but they don't make us feel better. In fact, we're much worse off after the effects wear off.

Here's an extreme example to illustrate the point:

Back when Charlie was fifteen, he had a really rough day in school. He failed his math test, the kids were making fun of him in class, and he wasn't picked for the ball game at recess. Walking home sad and dejected, a kid hanging out on the corner asked him what was wrong.

"I failed my math test, the kids were making fun of me and I didn't get picked in the game," he answered despondently. At that point, the kid on the corner pulled out a small baggie with white powder and a syringe, handed it to Charlie with a few instructions, and told him to use it in order to feel better.

Charlie didn't give it much thought, put it in his pocket, and continued sulking down the street. He arrived home, and his parents, immediately upon seeing his melancholy mood, asked him the same question.

"What's wrong, dear?"

He provided the same answer: "I failed my math test, the kids were making fun of me, and I didn't get picked in the game." But as he was explaining his turmoil to his parents, he decided to take out the baggie from his pants, followed the instructions from the kid on the corner, and proceeded to inject the contents into his arm – right in front of his parents no less.

Moments after removing the syringe, a half-broken smile emerged on his face and his eyes turned glassy and distant. "Wow, I feel better now," he uttered in a volume just louder than a whisper.

His parents were mortified – overcome with shock and disbelief. Why? Their son was no longer feeling sad. He was temporarily absolved of his anguish. Why wouldn't they condone such behavior?

Even though the answer is patently apparent, it's highly instructive to illuminate. The cost far outweighs the gain. Besides the addictive and deadly properties inherent in the substance – which in and of itself is enough to cause considerable concern – the act of self-medicating to sedate stress is destructive and debilitating, further seeding the sequence of escape and avoidance of seeking solutions.

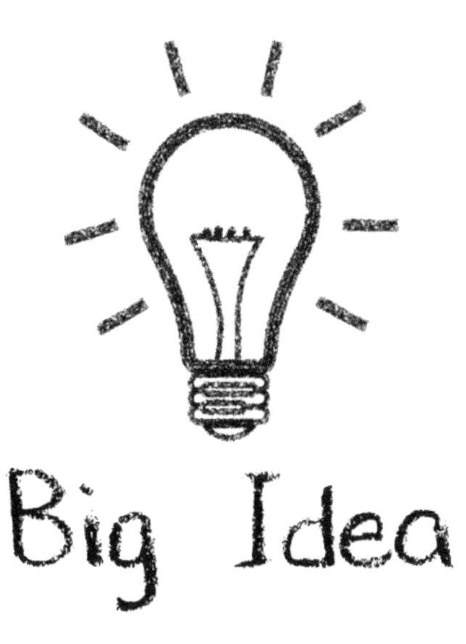

Running away from life's issues – whether with the aid of dangerous drugs, or the more mundane Milky Way bar -- is chasing the ultimate counterfeit pleasure. Our goal is not to feel good for the moment – no matter the consequence – but to release our stress in a productive manner that leaves us better off at the end, not worse off.

We're certainly not looking to be stoic soldiers, welcoming abuse with the famous refrain, "Thank you, sir, may I have another?" And we're not trying to solve the problem at that moment, but rather mitigate the temporary internal ache that arises as a result, without causing ourselves further harm.

I find it helpful to characterize stress as: emotional toxins. The symptoms resulting from a flu, cold or stomach virus – such as sneezing, perspiring, vomiting, or diarrhea -- are definitely not pleasant experiences to undergo, but they are nonetheless very valuable. It's our body's way of releasing toxins. It would be far, far worse if we were incapable of eliminating them from our system and they remained inside.

PURGE, DON'T PLUNGE

I believe the same parallel can be ascribed to anxiety, anger, and stress. Those are emotional toxins, as it were, that also need to be purged out instead of stuffed in. We are all aware of – and have probably experienced first-hand -- the stress-relief benefits achieved by exercise or venting to a friend. Having someone to talk to, or a physical activity in which to engage, doesn't necessarily resolve the core issue. It's not meant to.

But it serves the incredibly constructive function of exorcising that negative emotional energy.

Sports, walking, running, yoga, meditating, talking, and journaling are just some examples of highly useful and easily accessible vehicles of release. And here's the key point: We're always better off after the fact – unless you twist your ankle on the basketball court.

We didn't defeat the underlying dilemma, but we helped to recalibrate our emotional equilibrium. Stuffing down our feelings with an apple strudel, however, just adds to the angst as soon as the serotonin from the sugar subsides, leaving us with a hardened heart and bloated belly.

Purge, don't plunge. We need to purge our stress, not plunge it down with food.

Let's come back to Charlie, who just got his first job as a stock boy stacking loads of heavy boxes. He labors exhaustively but is empowered to push on by the thought of his first pay day. Friday finally arrives, he collects the envelope with five $100 bills as his first life earnings, and hurries to the bank to deposit his hard-earned wages.

He hands them to the teller with a proud smile, which quickly turns to a horrified frown when the teller swipes her brown marker over the bills and declares that they are counterfeit. Speechless and emotionally spent, he has absolutely nothing to show for his investment of time and energy. His sweat equity was worthless. He literally and figuratively is left empty-handed.

Every time we binge on biscuits and gravy, we end up

in the same despondent and demoralized place as Charlie, having pursed a counterfeit pleasure that left us with nothing more than remorse, regret, and clogged arteries. That certainly ain't no gravy train.

At this point I want to emphasize that by no means I am downplaying the dangers of drug use and the magnitude of the impact it has on our society. But we also have to be cognizant of the fact that more people die as a direct result of obesity than from all overdoses combined. It ranks second only behind smoking as the number one cause of preventable death in the United States. And the gap appears to be closing.

And even though we're soberly aware of the statistics, I don't believe we look at it through the same lenses. Perhaps we need to adjust this prescription as well. In fact, we see all around us that comfort foods are overtly, enthusiastically, and aggressively promoted. Competitive eating is a growing sport at the same time as weight gain and obesity are among the primary sources accounting for the skyrocketing cost of health care. Diabetes has been designated as the fastest-growing disease in the history of modern medicine.

Based on the feedback I've collected from the more than 1,000 clients I've worked with during the past decade, emotional eating is the top issue they identify as the cause of their weight problem and ongoing unhealthy habits.

And everyone wants to stop. But they approach it with

a fatal flaw. "Eli," they say. "I'll cut out the emotional eating if you can give me something in its place." That doesn't sound like an unreasonable request. Didn't we just speak about the value of positive actions and outlets to expel those emotional toxins?

Certainly.

But what if the situation arose that – for whatever reason – they were not able to quickly access one of those productive choices? Should their fallback be Fig Newtons?

Certainly not.

A vital ingredient critical in our recipe for recovery is the concept that our abstinence has to be intrinsic, not dependent. Abstaining from compulsive behaviors and emotional eating has to be a given in our mindset of commitment and resolve, not a laudatory accomplishment achieved only in an environment of ideal conditions. There are three compelling reasons upon which I base this conclusion.

1. For many of us, the forecast for rain in our emotional world is not infrequent and our busy and hectic lives don't always lend themselves toward immediately accessible constructive outlets.

2. Our muscle memory is to reach for the muffins when torment first starts tapping us on the back. That's been our default for so long and is such an ingrained reaction that if we give ourselves even the slightest possibility to choose

that option, our alignment will drift quickly toward that ditch.

We have to be willing to bear those five uncomfortable minutes – the time it takes for the intensity of the emotional anguish to stop boiling over. Sometimes five minutes extends into a half hour, but regardless, the only way toward breaking the habit is to no longer see it as a viable alternative, no matter what the circumstance.

Here we see the six-year-old syndrome surfacing again. Remember Sarah and her six-year-old niece Miriam from the broken roller coaster? They're coming home one night to a dark house caused by a temporary electrical outage. They enter the side door, feeling their way toward the coat closet, when they both stub their big toes on the couch that was moved to the middle of the room earlier in the day to look for a missing game.

The lights come back on and both Sarah and Miriam are now sitting on the couch but reacting very differently to their throbbing toes. Miriam, as you guessed, is wailing hysterically, while Sarah is rubbing her toe and grimacing. We ask the same question: Why are their reactions so different even though the pain is relatively equal?

Because Miriam, as a six-year-old, lives in the moment, and therefore her whole life is revolving around her current condition. She's panicking not so much from the pain but from the perception that it will never go away. Sarah has the benefit of perspective, absorbs those five uncomfortable minutes, and then moves on because she knows the pain will subside.

And what did Sarah do to comfort Miriam? She gave her a hug and a kiss, caressed her hair, and then an amazing thing occurred. Miriam ran off to play as if it never happened. Sarah helped change her emotional channel and refocus on the new and next five minutes of her life.

Now, it's never a bad thing to be comforted and caressed. But, as adults, we don't need that to get over a stubbed toe. We can absorb those five uncomfortable minutes until it stops smarting. That's the wise thing to do.

And that's why applying the wisdom of "This too shall pass" is so imperative in breaking the bonds of emotional eating. Stay on the bus, because the scenery will change. Our feelings are also fluid. We won't be caught in the ditch of despair unless we jump off the bus, because then we'll be stuck in that crummy neighborhood.

If we flail for food to assuage our anxiety, we'll "wake up" after those few minutes of momentary distraction reeling in the results of our rancid reaction. "I can't believe I did that again!"

Which brings us to the third reason, which by now should seem self-evident.

Would Charlie's parents respond this way? Would

they tell him to stop taking the drugs only on the condition that he finds a more appropriate means of pain avoidance? Of course not. Their cease and desist order is immediate and intrinsic, not dependent on accessing a better alternative.

They certainly want to help Charlie overcome his current emotional agony – but if there was no other option available at that moment, they would much prefer him to "ride out the waves of sadness" than get bitten by the shark in the syringe.

And on a broader scope, that's one of the skills we need to learn in our developmental change. It's okay to feel our feelings. It's never okay to feed them. Happy, mad, glad, or sad are emotional states in which we all reside at some time or another – sometimes in the same day, and sometimes even simultaneously in more than one. It doesn't mean we're schizophrenic, just human.

We can all muster the courage to face our stuff and not stuff our face if we maintain the clarity of consequence and the belief in the benefit. We can accept ourselves as wonderful yet imperfect people progressing through life and acting precisely with our food plan.

We can realize that the power inside of us is always stronger than the problem in front of us. And if we are of a spiritual nature, then the Power above us is certainly greater than the problem in front of us.

Which dovetails to what I believe is the core cure for the source of much of our stress and emotional discomfort: learning how to no longer fan the flames of frustration.

The feeling of frustration spontaneously combusts when filling the gap between expectation and reality.

When we project unrealistic expectations on another person – especially a close relative or friend -- and they come up short in our eyes, our resulting reaction is often one of anger and frustration. This ignites an emotional fire that burns inside of us and our rapid response is to turn toward food to douse the flames – a chocolate milkshake being the ultimate fire retardant.

The flip side of frustration is fueled by what we think we can control versus what is actually in our hands to change – which, I hate to break it to you, is nothing more than ourselves. Like we spoke about regarding the attitude of Necessity in the chapter on the key of C.H.A.N.G.E., it's not a contradiction to live with the reality that while we have awesome roles to play and responsibilities to fill in regard to others, the only person we have singular control over is ourselves.

So, therefore, you're the only one that you can change. Power down your projected expectations on others and unleash the incredible power you have inside yourself to meet your remarkable potential.

I'm not saying that as some pop psychologist, rank cheerleader, or "the glass is half full kind of guy."

I live with the resolute understanding that no human being is vestigial. No one is born without some purpose or meaning in life. I've never met a talking tonsil or appendix – even though I have neither. Every person has some ability to make a magnificent impact on this world. We can surely change others primarily by concentrating on maximizing our unique capabilities.

I'm convinced that this concept is the among the most effective vaccines to inoculate ourselves from the disease of emotional turmoil and the subsequent intense inclination many of us have for the antidote of comfort food.

We can encapsulate it in the following formula: surrender equals serenity. Allow me to define the term. Surrender doesn't mean giving in, and it certainly doesn't mean giving up. It means giving it over. We need to give over emotional control of those things – and people – about which we have no control.

The more we accept the things we cannot change (others) and focus on changing the things we can (ourselves) the more emotional serenity we'll develop, and the less disposed we'll be toward emotional eating.

As someone brilliantly summarized:

"A good day is when everything goes right and I do not binge. A great day is when nothing goes right and I do not binge."

I wish everyone only a good day today. But if you must, then make it a great day.

"Thank you for all you have done in helping me this year. I realize it comes from inside me, but I could not have found what I needed to without your guidance. I am finishing the year over thirty pounds lighter than last year and feeling like a completely different and healthy person. My food choices have changed dramatically, as has the way I see food and eating. I still have much work to do, but I have made so much more progress than I ever thought I could."

- Marc, Baltimore, Maryland

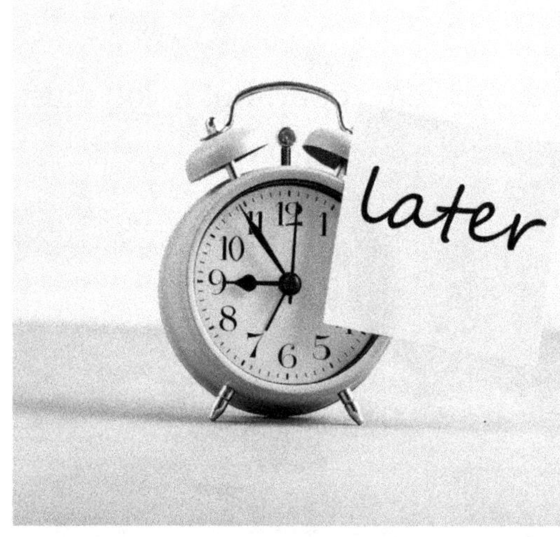

9

KEY FIVE: TODAY IS THE CURE FOR THE DISEASE OF TOMORROW

"Don't worry, I'll get back on my diet tomorrow."

"Tomorrow, I'm absolutely going to join the gym."

"First thing tomorrow I'll to go to the store and buy that new weight-loss book."

Tomorrow, tomorrow, tomorrow.

We have all lived through a lifetime of tomorrows, and

where did that get us? With nothing more than a year full of empty yesterdays.

We use the "disease" of tomorrow as a promising pillow of procrastination on which to rest our raging rationalizations, giving us solace to succumb to our immediate inclinations – even though it will end up being nothing more than an agonizing bed of nails.

We're not inherently untrustworthy people. But we have a genuine talent for being internally disingenuous when it comes to justifying a palatable passion. The Bible may be mankind's most read book, but substantiating spontaneous succulence is perhaps the planet's most penned manuscript. And it's an ever-growing work in progress – and no doubt one of the leading causes for the pandemic of worldwide obesity.

That's why unconditional honesty is one of the fundamental principles to which I keep circling back. Long-term weight loss is not about sacrifice or starvation or being strong or strict – and it's certainly not about waiting for tomorrow's newest miracle diet. It's about the willingness to be unconditionally honest with ourselves and our feelings about food. To admit that we are respectable people with a remarkable penchant to be self-deceiving when it comes to defending a dietary desire.

It's one of the indispensable moving parts that we must manage as we engage in this transformative process. It's about recognizing that this is our intellectual predisposition in our relationship with food and therefore understanding that our daily duties are to develop and sustain an awareness of objective honesty to counterbalance our tendency toward subjective reasoning.

We have to continually compensate for our chronic misalignment in order not to drift into the ditch. And just like riding a bike, maintaining this equilibrium is not excruciatingly difficult, but essential nevertheless.

And that's why I call it the "disease" of tomorrow. It's dis-eased thinking – a dearth of direct and deliberate discernment when confronted with a desire for a Danish.

A second, and just as maddening manifestation of the "disease" of tomorrow is the fear of the future.

"You mean I can't have pizza for the rest of my life?!"

"How can I be expected to stick to my food plan during summer vacation?!"

"It's going to take me forever to lose 100 pounds!"

We're projecting the consequences of our current commitment on to the coming days, weeks, months, or years and conclude that we're incapable of that level of consistency.

Right now, we may be perfectly resolute in our intellectual recognition and internal acceptance that lasagna is a liability, not an asset in achieving our inviolable priority of losing weight and changing our relationship with food. Our head and heart are aligned. We're good with it.

But then our eyes begin peering up from above our daily plate of immediate aspirations and start gazing into the future and the perceived potential pitfalls – based either on the longevity required to meet our goal or the challenging environments or temptations with which we'll be confronted. Suddenly, our unbendable commitment becomes highly pliable. Our firm foundation has faded to a weak-kneed posture.

What happened?

We invest our emotional energy into the fear of the future, which paralyzes us from being successful in the present. Our determination account, which was just flush with purpose and resolve, is now teetering on bankruptcy. We've been robbed of our willingness by a con man masquerading as reasonable expectations. And the tragedy is that it was all an inside job. That stinking thinking sank us again.

But there is an antidote. It's called TODAY. Today is the cure for the disease of tomorrow – and thus the next of the Seven Soveya Keys to unlock our blocks.

"Tired and trite," may be your first reaction. "Tried and true," is my resounding response.

Let's explain.

There's absolutely nothing wrong with thinking ahead and preparing for the future – whether financially, for our career, family, or any other important aspect of our life. It'd be pretty laborious and burdensome to continually shop for only one day's worth of groceries.

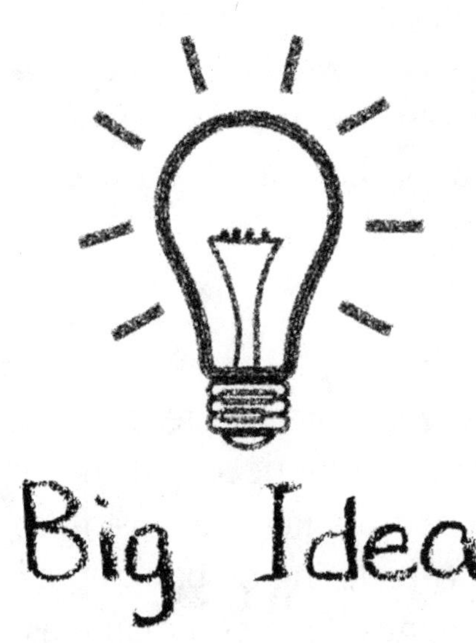

The disease of the tomorrow is not the exercise of planning for the future. That's responsible and mature. The disease of tomorrow is the perception that ***today*** we need to possess the strength and acuity to bear the burden of successfully fulfilling our future accomplishments. That's the major misconception to which we fall prey -- which quickly creates a feeling of doubt and uncertainty about even possessing the capability to succeed in the present.

Why is this such an enormous error?

Because upon waking up each morning, we're all gifted with an emotional reservoir of energy to supply us just for that day – to undertake those tasks and engage those challenges that color our calendar and appear on our path. Our head may strategize over a 12-month span, but we need to keep the schedule in our heart locked on the daily view. Understandable anxiety impulsively ignites if we envision our shoulders supporting the weight of all our future endeavors.

It's faulty math. Our emotional account is not meant to fund a year's worth of withdrawals – just like the water reservoir supplying New York City is not designed to meet the demands of Philadelphia as well.

If we have the resolution to refrain from a root-beer float for today, that's the singular intention upon which we need to direct our emotional energy. Worrying about how we're going to "hold ourselves back" from partaking in pasta for the rest of our lives is a woefully misplaced concern. It's completely irrelevant and fundamentally counterproductive to the objective at hand – which is to keep our hands off the noodles just for those next several hours until hitting the pillow that night.

And then an amazing thing happens the following morning. Our reservoir is restocked with a sufficient supply of emotional currency to spend for that next day. That's one of the incredible functions of sleep. It allows us to reframe, refocus, re-energize, and recharge. It's a daily direct deposit in our determination account. We can regain the clarity of our conviction and the mental consensus that we're capable of keeping to our commitments and possess the wherewithal to withstand any temptations that may develop during the day.

In this case, kicking the can down the road is entirely encouraged and a great use of our feet. For here is one of the prophetic guarantees I'm going to share in the pages of this book: Neither you, nor I – nor anyone – knows for certain how we will feel tomorrow. Our commitment may be concrete, or it may be compromised. We simply have no idea. We're not there.

I hate to break it to you, but we have no time machine nor predictive powers to accurately ascertain the degree of our future fortitude and mental makeup. So, why in the world would we allow a mindset about which we have no clue inform and guide our attitude today?

"But I've failed so many times in the past," you may say. Your dieting history hints loudly to an inability to maintain sustained success. Point well taken. However, there are two important differences that we must consider.

Firstly, I would hazard to surmise that the vast majority of your previous attempts were focused on changing your weight, and not on changing yourself and relationship with food. As we've seen up to this point, that is a formula for failure and a recipe for relapse. It's the Band-Aid approach to healing a chronic infection.

Secondly, just like the classic disclaimer of financial investment is "Past success does not guarantee future performance," the flip side is also true: "Previous collapses don't ensure future failures." None of us are doomed to dietary disaster, no matter our past experience. That's not only the premise of the Soveya Solution, it's the evidence I've personally encountered and witnessed for the past fifteen years.

Taking it one day at a time is the only express train with the best chance of getting you to your destination on time. And what I can safely say with confident conviction is that if tomorrow you employ the same tools and take the same actions that produced a healthy and productive relationship with food today, there's a darn good chance you'll get the same results. And that's the conveyor belt of consistency upon which the Soveya Solution progresses – a daily exercise in keeping our head and heart in the right place so our hands will execute the right choices.

It has nothing to do with weight loss or dieting. That's why I emphasize these ideas until I'm blue in the face – or in the case of this book, blue in the fingers. Long-term success is nothing more than an accumulation of daily accomplishments. That's all it is – and that's everything it is: Maintaining the willingness to be proactive in managing our mindset and emotional welfare in our relationship with food – JUST FOR TODAY.

And the first intake of fuel that powers our daily engine of resolve is called <u>The Three Reinforcements</u>. There's no better way to launch the day than with this high-octane starter fluid. If, soon after arising, we dutifully digest these three doctrines, we will provide an invaluable reinforcement to our daily dedication.

1). ***We didn't regret it!*** If we prioritized our health, stuck to our food plan, and maintained our boundaries irrespective of what yesterday threw at us, we never look back the next morning and say, "You know what, I really wish I would have had the cannoli instead of the cantaloupe." If we keep our mouth away from the macaroons, those words will never cross our lips and our daily journey will continually cross the finish line of success.

We never regret doing the right thing, making the appropriate choices and investing our time and effort into achieving our goals. In contrast to the countless times we awoke awash in the inner shame and sorrow of having blown it again – all for a sorry serving of sweet and sour chicken.

2). ***We feel good!*** What a concept! Waking up ***not*** feeling bloated, gaseous, distended and disheartened. We actually feel good physically – and feel good about ourselves. Our body is working optimally because we didn't overrun it with onion rings. We treated it with respect and are infused with the integrity that inevitably follows a day filled with healthy, balanced meals. That's way more rewarding than any fortune cookie.

3). ***It wasn't as hard as we thought!*** Here's the knockout punch – or in our case, the galvanizing kick in the pants. So many times, our momentary subjective fears massage a manageable molehill into a massive mountainside, convincing us that we have no choice but to detour directly to the donuts. We can't deal with this emotional turmoil without a quick fix of fried dough, or planning and carrying out our food plan is too taxing and time consuming with everything else going on right now that we have to deviate from our plan and improvise with ice cream.

That's the landscape as seen through our faulty vision. We become paralyzed by our perception instead of fueled by facts. That's because the *perception* of the degree of difficulty is 99% of the time greater than the *actual* degree of difficulty. It's not as hard as we think. We really can carry out our plan in the face of everything else going on around us. The requisite amount of mental focus and faith in ourselves fuels our feet to keep taking one step forward throughout the day, instead of getting mired in the mud of misperception.

And upon waking up the next morning, having walked through our fears the day before instead of being floored by them, we jump to the ceiling with delight and an uber clarity that it wasn't nearly as onerous as our mental screenwriter envisioned. The coming attractions weren't so accurate after all. Gee, go figure.

We need to actively take stock of these three reinforcements each morning in order to enrich our account. It doesn't necessarily happen by osmosis. It's not such heavy lifting, and we'll find that if we do the mental curls, we'll have copious amounts of emotional capital to divest and conquer that day's concerns.

And this strength training produces compound interest. For the more often we apply the key of TODAY in our daily eating encounters, we'll tellingly transform our entire outlook and relationship with food so when we do get to the summer vacation, we'll be in a distinctly different mindset to deal with the dilemma. For, in fact, it might not be such a dilemma at all, but rather just a series of actions that we're more than comfortable and committed to take in order to replicate our success and represent our ongoing priority of self-care through proper nourishment – no matter what environment in which we find ourselves.

This is the underlying basis for the answer I give when asked, "Eli, are you going to do this for the rest of your life?"

"I can't tell you what I'm going to do tomorrow because I'm still stuck in today. But I certainly plan on making the same decisions as I made yesterday, because those served me quite well and I have no reason to believe they won't produce the same results." I'm a big believer in: <u>if it ain't broke, don't fix it</u>.

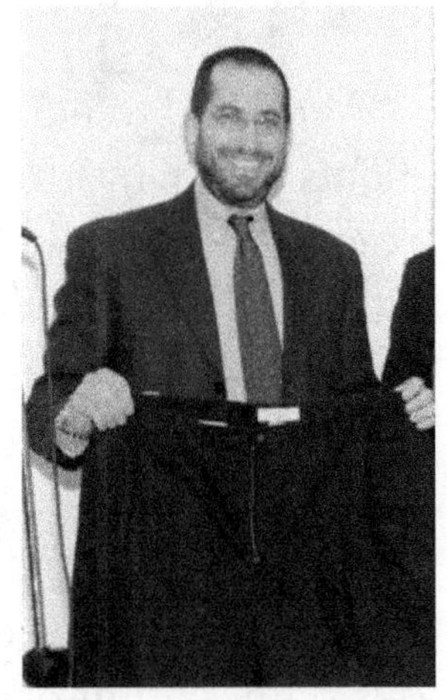

What are the dividends of my investment? What have I gained from learning to use food to meet my body's needs instead of indulging my desires? I lost 130 pounds and have remained within an ideal weight range for more than a decade and a half. I flipped the numbers in my BMI score (body mass index) from a morbidly obese 42 to a healthy 24. My pants went down 12 sizes.

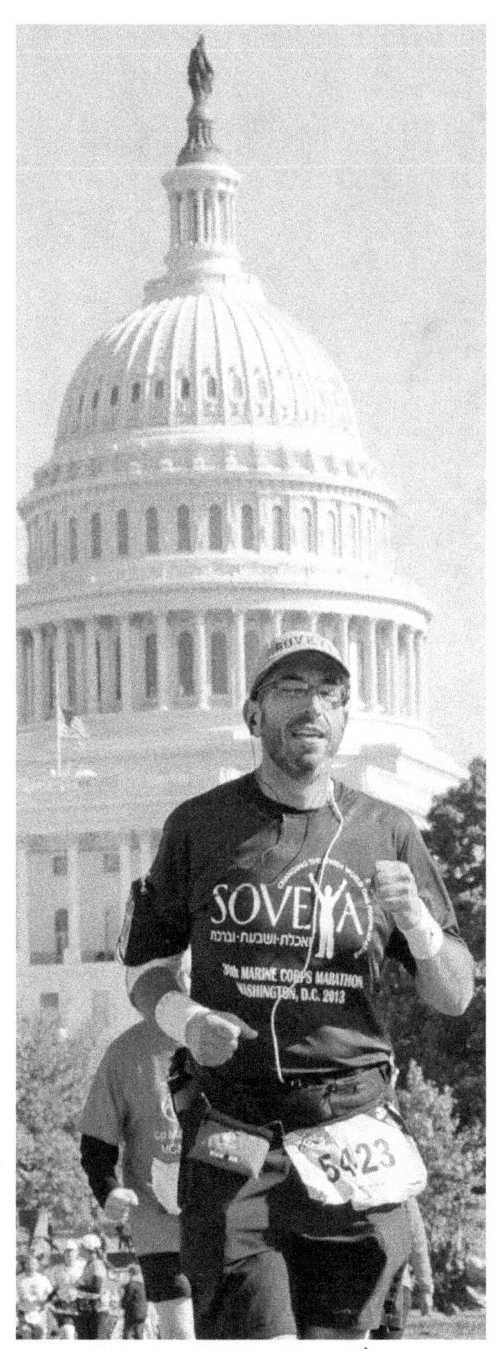

Marine Corps Marathon

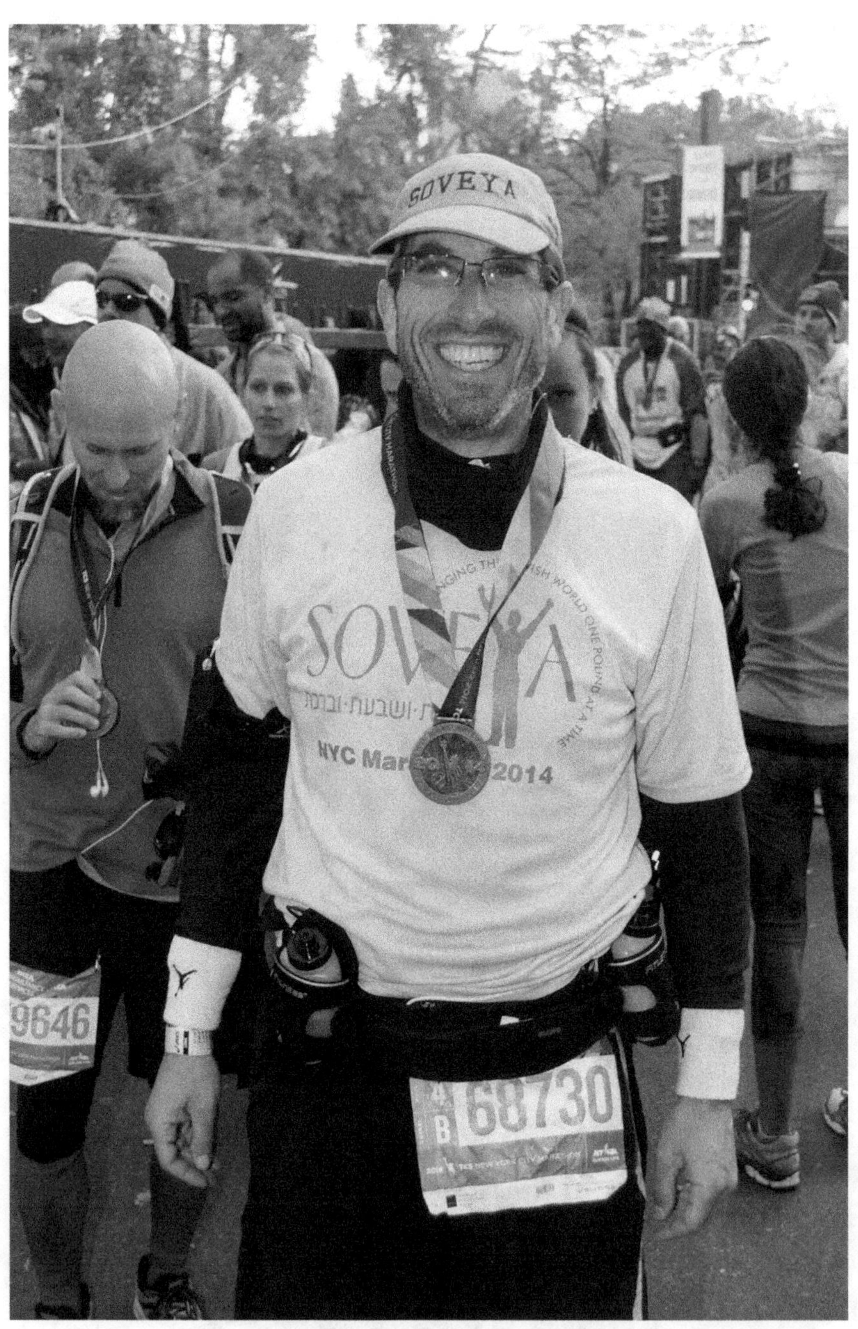

New York City Marathon

I've run countless marathons, half marathons, and 10K races and am in the best shape in my life. And most importantly, I lost the 1,000 pounds or regret and remorse off of my shoulders as a result of my freedom from food obsession. I'm doing everything in my control to provide a healthy father for my children and husband for my wife.

During the past seventeen years, I can say with unwavering clarity that I have never regretted any choices I made that continued to build and bolster my abstinence. They have always left me physically and emotionally in a better place than the alternative. And they really weren't that overwhelmingly oppressive – to say the least.

This is the goal for the future that we can all set today. To have the ability, desire, and self-worth to make the decisions that are distinctively right for us – one day at a time. To treat food as fuel for our body and strive to meet our guidelines of Q.Q.T. – Quality, Quantity, and Timing. That's the framework of what the right decision will look like even if we don't know what the exact technical details will be. If we plan to take care of our food plan, the food plan will take care of us.

And if we stay in the day, the abstinence will stay in us.

"Thank you so much for your encouragement, support, and belief in me (even when I fall, you believe that I can get up and continue working on myself to have a healthy relationship with food, day by day). I am on the plan, really feeling great, energized, and busy with other things, not solely food. I feel accomplished, purposeful, confident, in the moment, and not worried about what the future may bring."

– Rebecca, Lakewood, New Jersey

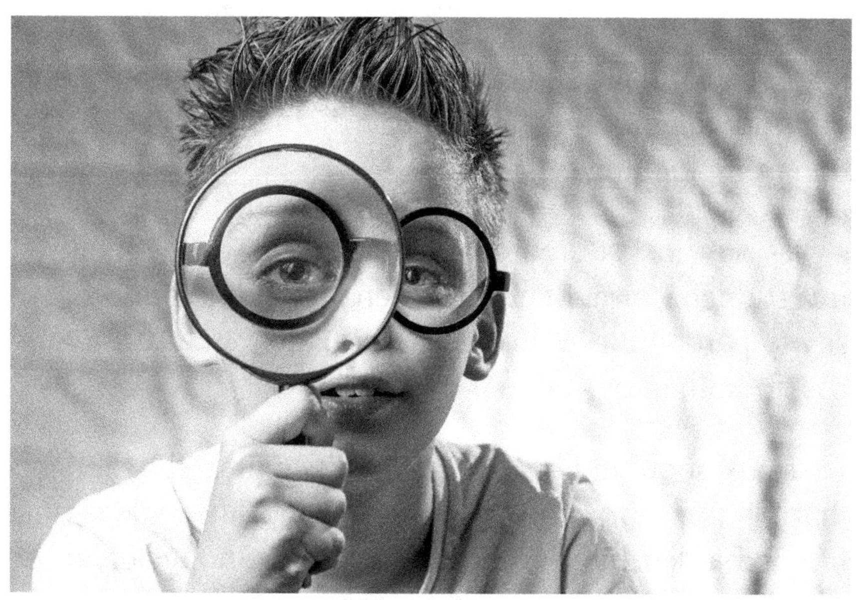

10

KEY SIX: CLARITY IS KEY

Clarity. As you have probably figured out by now, this word ranks among the highest entries in the Soveya dictionary. It should be indelibly etched in our mental hard drive. We can't leave home without it.

Just like when traveling to Paris, we're literally tongue-tied and basically immobile without our pocket-sized English-French translation guide (or nowadays, the vocabulary app on our mobile device), so too when we enter any challenging food environment, our success is severely handicapped if we don't have a firm hold on our clarity. It's the sweatband around our wrists that keeps us from losing our grip, and across our forehead that keeps the perspiration from flooding our eyes.

It's our pocket umbrella that keeps us from getting wet in a sudden storm. Because, when it comes to our propensity to pardon a piece of pecan pie, there's always a forecast for rain in our brain.

Think about it. Let's compare and contrast the thoughts that occupy our headspace before and after taking that first forbidden bite. We'll call it the forethought and the afterthought. The forethought is the mental gymnastics we so eloquently execute to excuse the éclair. Our aptitude to appease our conscience and cloud our clarity when confronted with a can of caramel corn is incredible. We lose sight of our sound judgment and let our lucidity lapse through our slippery fingers.

As we saw in the previous chapter of The Disease of Tomorrow, we can formulate any number of "valid" reasons to rationalize our momentary desire. "It's okay – just this time. I'll be fine. It's so delicious, I have to taste just one. What's the big deal?" That's the forethought.

But how do we feel afterwards? No sooner do we polish off the last bite then we are pained with the somber reality that, "It **wasn't** okay. I didn't need to eat that. I would have been fine without it. I can't believe I did it again."

Those two thoughts are diametrically opposed. They aren't 179 degrees apart – they are 180 degrees opposite. One is demonstrably true, and one is fundamentally false. Care to guess which is which?

You got it! The afterthought is the objective reality while the forethought is the subjective justification. So the million-dollar question is, how do we maintain the clarity of the afterthought ***at the time*** of the forethought?

And thus we're introduced to the next of the Seven Soveya Keys – aptly named the Clarity List.

It's a simple document that could simply spell the difference between success and failure. Consequences and Benefits. By creating a chart and populating these two columns, we give ourselves the ability to see clearly and stay in our lane when the rain begins to fog our windshield and reduce our visibility.

We've all had those what I call "two-in-the-morning" moments. We're lying in bed and staring at the ceiling saturated with the sober certainty of how our unhealthy eating habits have affected our lives. We're done for the day trying to fool others – or ourselves. No more games or excuses. In our pitch-black bedroom, we possess the ultimate clarity that as good as the chocolate cake tastes – *IT'S JUST NOT WORTH IT*!

Whereas when it was on our plate, our vision was locked in to the confines of the four square inches of fudge-covered cake, we now can see beyond the last bite, and all the crumbs of crummy consequences that predictably trail behind. The sincerity of this insight may energize us enough to take an action toward change, but often doesn't propel us beyond the next few days, if not even the next couple of waking hours – where we find ourselves once again confounded, confused and quickly copping the cupcakes.

What happened to our clarity of the consequences? The brilliance of that light lasted as long as the lightning bolt. And our mistake was relying on that flash of light to change us instead of merely showing direction. We have to take the steps – and that starts with capturing that clarity and housing it in our hand-held flashlight, which we need to manually turn on and illuminate our path each day. Because when it comes to our relationship with food, our honesty power plant often suffers random blackouts.

Always be prepared.

Two distinct memories I have of my wonderful cousin Sylvia, of blessed memory, were her collection of hundreds of miniature porcelain turtles positioned all around her apartment, and the tightly folded tissue she always had neatly tucked inside the cuff of her sweater, ready at any moment to be unleashed from under her right wrist. Because you never know when you might need to suddenly blow your nose.

The Clarity List should be just as accessible – and I'm not exaggerating.

As you see on the corresponding chart, the Clarity List catalogues the Consequences – both physical and emotional – resulting from our unhealthy eating habits. Be thorough and exhaustive when filling it out. Don't hold anything back. Exercise the same diligence on the Benefits side. What are the positive effects of having a healthy and wholesome relationship with food? They can either be the inverse of many of the consequences, or independent values as well. Treat it as a "working document," meaning be ready and willing to add entries to the lists as the ideas come to mind.

SOVEYA
WEIGHT LOSS SOLUTION

CLARITY LIST

CONSEQUENCES	BENEFITS
HEALTH: high blood pressure; high cholesterol; heart disease; diabetes; stroke; cancer; shortened life span; difficulty getting pregnant; joint problems; fatty liver syndrome; gallbladder disease; increased risks to mother and baby at child birth; higher chance for miscarriage.	**HEALTH**: longer life; reversal of type 2 diabetes; reduced risk of cardiovascular disease; normal blood pressure; healthy cholesterol levels; easier to conceive and give birth; less chance of premature labor; less pressure on joints and bones.
CONDITIONS & SYMPTOMS: sleep apnea; gout; shortness of breath; hard to walk & climb stairs; back pain; knee pain; lack of energy/always tired; snoring; restless sleeping; a lot of medications; continually checking blood sugar; CPAP machine so cumbersome to sleep with and have to schlep it whenever I travel.	**CONDITIONS & SYMPTOMS**: more energy; feel healthy and fit; easier to breath; no pain in back or knees; easier to walk, exercise and play with kids (or grandkids); not falling asleep at dinner table; few or no medications; improved intimacy; easier to travel; better able to take care of physical responsibilities and strenuous chores.
EMOTIONAL & PSYCHOLOGICAL: depression; low self-esteem; stress; hate the way I look; lack of patience; short tempered; lack of control; slave to my desires; constantly obsessing or thinking about food; ongoing regret and shame; feel like a failure.	**EMOTIONAL & PSYCHOLOGICAL**: feel better about myself; in a good mood; more patience with family and friends; feel attractive and like the way I look in clothes; freedom from food obsession; not controlled by my cravings; freer mind to think about more important things; self-confidence; personal integrity; feel tremendous satisfaction in overcoming this challenge.
PERSONAL, FAMILY & SOCIETY: bad example for my children; not attractive to my spouse; lack of credibility in eyes of others; harder to find a job; harder to find dates; hypocritical to be overweight health-care provider or spiritual leader; can't fit into my clothes; need seat-belt extender; self-conscious & embarrassed at social events; isolate a lot; can't shop in regular stores; cost of prescriptions or diabetes meds; higher premiums or difficulty getting life insurance.	**PERSONAL, FAMILY & SOCIETY**: spouse finds me appealing; good example for family; more credibility and value in workplace; feel confident in social settings; not afraid of showing up to group events; comfortable in my own skin; saving money on fewer medication costs and insurance premiums; more mobile and flexible to travel; ready to learn and try new things in life; willing to step out of my comfort zone.

At the same time, don't make it complicated. No prose required. Just a concise yet comprehensive list of key words or phrases that will generate sudden sobriety – or even more importantly, will serve as secure investments in your clarity account and honesty holdings. Because you never know when you might need to make a withdrawal.

Focus on the flu shot.

Utilizing this key as a flu shot is much more effective and impactful than merely trying to rely on it as an antibiotic. For the sake of clarity and full disclosure (apropos for this chapter) this following comparison is not meant to condemn or condone flu shots or antibiotics or render any medical advice. It's simply proffered to posit what I believe is a very poignant point by means of illustration.

Steven has been sick for a little while and doesn't seem to be getting any better. He finally goes to his doctor, who diagnoses him with a bacterial infection and prescribes antibiotics to facilitate his healing. Seems like a reasonable course of action. Steven is already symptomatic and is taking medicine to help him get better.

Sandra, on the other hand, goes to the pharmacy with her niece Susan to get a flu shot. As the pharmacist sticks the needle in her arm, Susan looks up at her aunt and asks, "You're not sick; why is he giving you medicine?" A great question.

Sandra answers, "You're right, Susan. I feel great now. But in a few weeks there will be a lot of germs in the air and it will be easier for someone to get sick, so I'm taking this medicine today to help protect my body from the viruses that will probably be around beginning next month."

What's the main difference between the two?

Steven is already symptomatic and is being reactive. Sandra is not yet symptomatic and being proactive to help prevent the problem in the first place.

Once we are triggered with a craving, it's much harder to first start building up our emotional immune system on the spot when already confronted with the cheesecake. Bearing any previous preparations, we certainly want to try and reach for the raft of reason and rationality when we fear falling overboard. But our sea-legs are already wobbly and our balance is less than stable. It's like trying to affix the storm shutters to our windows when the winds have already reached gale-force strength. It's usually a losing battle.

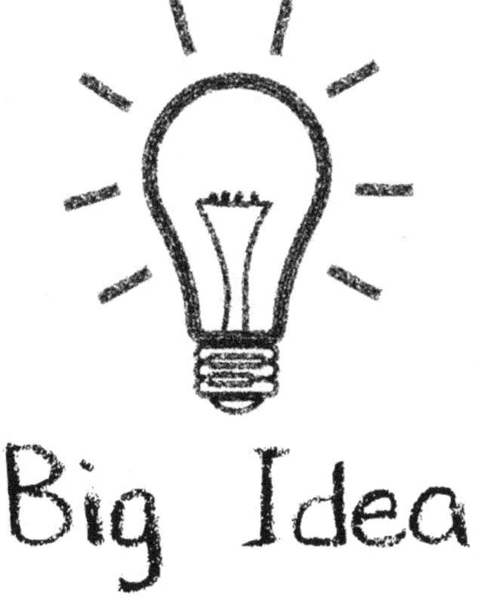

We need to take our flu shots *before* we're compromised. We need to go to Home Depot, get our boards and nails, and put up the shutters while it's still sunny. The calm before the storm is when the successful preparations take place.

When does that translate for us? Usually, right

after finishing the meal on our Soveya Food Plan. We're satisfied, satiated, and content in the knowledge that we robustly nourished ourselves and have sufficient fuel in our body to energize us until our next meal. We feel fine and are asymptomatic – which is the ideal time to make a deposit in our clarity account and reinforce our honest holdings.

The next few hours might be smooth sailing under a bright blue sky in our continuing journey of healthy eating, or an unexpected emotional weather front may rapidly rear in our radar – which many times isn't so unforeseen after all.

Or it could simply be a case like our friend, Rob, who was busy at work without obsessing over food until his co-worker walks in with the pizza, which trips Rob's rapid-response-rationalization wires. His cravings and mental commotion shoot off the starting line from zero to 60 in under five seconds.

The Clarity List helps keeps his hands firmly on the parking brake and off the ignition switch.

Here's how it works: Immediately upon finishing our food after each meal, we take a deep breath and read both sides of the list out loud--not necessarily loud enough for others to hear, but with enough energy and volume to engage our attention and prevent us from just skimming it over with our eyes. We then recite the following declaration: "I commit that nothing, absolutely nothing, will go in my mouth between now and my next meal. And I will not only survive, I'll thrive." You can announce that to another person if you like, or just say it to yourself. But don't avoid this affirmation.

We're actually training ourselves to fast between meals – what a revelation! -- to learn to live life between one meal and the next without the ever-present possibility of grazing, noshing, bingeing, or grabbing. We're not going to panic at those first pangs of hunger or lash out when lured by those first loops of licorice.

Well, that's not entirely true, because not only can we consume water, seltzer, or tea (and coffee if you must) – we should go out of our way to hydrate. Drinking water between meals is an integral tool to help prolong our satiation and stabilize our blood sugar, giving us the physical foundation to support our commitment.

The Clarity List continually creates a fresh platform of honesty and objectivity upon which to accurately assess the cost of deviating from our food plan. It gives us the ability to see the crumbs which inevitably emanate from the cake – and how they directly and undoubtedly cause the perpetuation of the consequences and further the blocking of the benefits.

How can just a one-time caving in to the cream pie possibly prolong our high blood pressure, alarming cholesterol levels, sinking self-esteem or any of the other multitude of misfortunes that unwelcomingly reside on the consequences side of our list?

The answer is simple. None of us just woke up one morning ending up on the end-line of our despair. I didn't gain 130 pounds overnight. For me, for you – and for all of us – the consequences on our personal Clarity Lists are a culmination of hundreds, if not thousands of choices we made that fed our feeding frenzy and perpetuated our problematic relationship with food. It's a direct chain of events that spans the course of time. And each occasion we repeat those actions, we're directly extending the effects and obstructing the recovery – as well as our arteries.

Because it's not about the momentary caloric intake or lack of nutritional value. It has nothing to do with counting points or calculating ketosis. It's all about changing our behavior. And succumbing to this "one-time" impulse just continues to pump the heartbeat of our compulsion.

Therefore, at the time of the trigger, we're not trying to create this awareness from scratch – but rather lean on the wall of unconditional honesty that we erected and reinforced just a short time ago upon engaging and internalizing the Clarity List. That freshly fashioned resolve and crisp commitment can serve to counterbalance the craving and confusion churning inside of us. Our bright and bold boundaries are on the forefront of our mind, allowing us to maintain the clarity of the afterthought at the time of the forethought. We're securely tethered to the truth while tempted with the tiramisu.

The flu shot doesn't dissipate the virus, it just guards us from being infected. The umbrella doesn't clear away the clouds, it just protects us from getting wet. So too, the Clarity List doesn't disintegrate the donuts, it just helps us dispel the notion that it's too hard, too uncomfortable, too tempting, or too depriving to do without.

We don't have to lose our mind and submit to the temporary insanity. We can turn our nose up at that stinking thinking that used to saturate our soul with the foul smell of remorse and regret. Our vulnerability no longer has to equate inevitability.

If we humbly acknowledge and enthusiastically accept that we need this thrice-daily dose of determination, we'll gladly invest the time and effort to religiously stick to our prescription – which will keep our perception pristine and our choices in concert with our goals and priorities, not in conflict.

There will always be viruses in our environment. That's a fact of life. Our susceptibility when it comes to food doesn't suspend us from the class of quality people in this world. No one walking this earth is free from some sort of subjective rationalization and improper inclinations. Our greatness is not based on the raw materials imbedded in us from our nature and nurture. It's all about the product we produce – because we're all works in progress.

And one of the keys to the key of the Clarity List is the recognition that it's really not such heaving lifting at all. It will probably take you all of 30 seconds – if that – to purposefully and punctiliously probe the Benefits and

Consequences, culminating with the two-sentence verbal declaration. That half-minute of investment will pay palpable dividends during the next few hours of your day and will certainly serve as your most satisfying dessert after every breakfast, lunch, and dinner.

"A number of years ago I worked with you and lost over thirty pounds. I have kept most of it off through eating sensibly. I have not had one cookie or sugary treat since I started working with you. My cholesterol and blood pressure are normal thanks to my new way of eating. Thanks for sending me in the right direction."

– Debbie, Miami, Florida

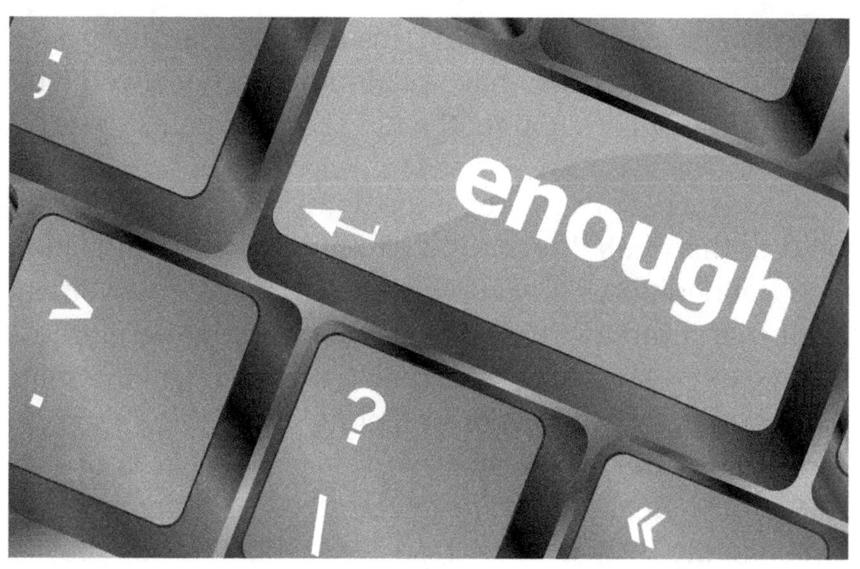

11

KEY SEVEN: ENOUGH IS ENOUGH

This phrase really captures the true essence of our transformation. For if you're willing to double down on both sides of this axiom, then you can truly transform the burden of saying "no" into the freedom to say "no" and create an enduring reformation in your relationship with food.

"Enough of this, already!" It begins with a genuine commitment sourced from uncompromising despair. Are you sick and tired of being sick and tired? Have you had enough of the endless bingeing and repeated returns to the starting line of a dieting journey that seems to grow more onerous, overwhelming, and insurmountable after each failed attempt? Do you have platinum status in a frequent-flyer club in which you loathe being a lifetime member?

Can you dig down deep enough into your soul and grab hold of that brutally raw and excruciating self-realization – to unconditionally acknowledge the most inconvenient truth that a mutiny upon the captain of your weight-loss voyage (Mr. Quick Fix) is the only remedy to right the ship? Are you finally ready to stop dieting and willing to go to **any lengths necessary** to reform and re-create your eating habits? Because, quite frequently, the difference between being 99% willing and 100% willing is not 1%, it's 1,000%, for the first step of real change often requires a giant leap of faith in yourself. Are you willing to take that first step and cast yourself as the lead role in your personalized production of Extreme Makeover?

Sounds too visceral and verbose? Is it any more extreme than spending hundreds of hours, thousands of dollars, and countless tears investing in another guaranteed, surefire, miracle diet that plays to your desperation by promoting a new-found formula for the fastest fat-burning program ever discovered? Can we permanently suspend our poisonous practice of perpetually suspending our disbelief for the blind faith of another can't-miss solution?

Are you ready to throw open the windows and shout from the rooftops, "I'M NOT GOING TO TAKE IT ANY MORE! ENOUGH IS FINALLY ENOUGH!" If so, then you're halfway there. Not halfway toward your goal weight, but midway toward an even more important destination: the firm ground of a foundational change of attitude and behavior that can support and sustain your daily transformation.

Some people change when they see the light. Most people change when they feel the heat. Have you had enough of being burnt by a torch bearing a single set of fingerprints – yours? If so, you want to convert this consummate clarity into the daily double of dedications called: "**whatever it takes**" and "**no matter what**."

Engage in this self-dialogue soon after arising in the morning. Ask yourself, "What am I going to do today to stick to my food plan and have a healthy relationship with food?" then answer unequivocally, "WHATEVER IT TAKES! Regardless of the cost involved, I'm worth investing in my health and wellbeing. Regardless of the effort required, I'm worth prioritizing my needs. Regardless of the challenges or emotional triggers that may arise, I don't have to use food to numb my feelings. NO MATTER WHAT, I'm going to maintain my dignity and self-respect, today. NO MATTER WHAT, I'm not going to hurt myself with food!"

"ENOUGH IS ENOUGH!"

And enough is in fact enough. The flipside of this coin is learning the A,B,Cs of "enough" – the three-stage emotional overhaul of our fear of being hungry or constrained. One of the first questions we ask about any new diet is, "Are there any foods that I can eat as much as I want?" "Can I at least have unlimited vegetables? What's free? Is there one 'cheat' food, or 'off' day with which I can treat myself?"

We have such a palpable fear of feeling restricted. Our association with eating and impulsivity is intoxicating. We feel so burdened to have to say "no" to ourselves. We're so boxed-in by boundaries that we're ready to burst.

A significant segment of the weight-loss industry is built on this premise. The all-you-can eat protein fad feeds this phobia. Diet-induced ketosis may help to stimulate temporary weight loss, but it certainly isn't a recipe for developing a long-term healthy and sustainable relationship with food. Why? Because we have to accept that enough really is enough. We must acknowledge that putting limits on our eating habits is not a necessary evil – but necessarily enabling. It's the only way we can manifest and maintain our makeover.

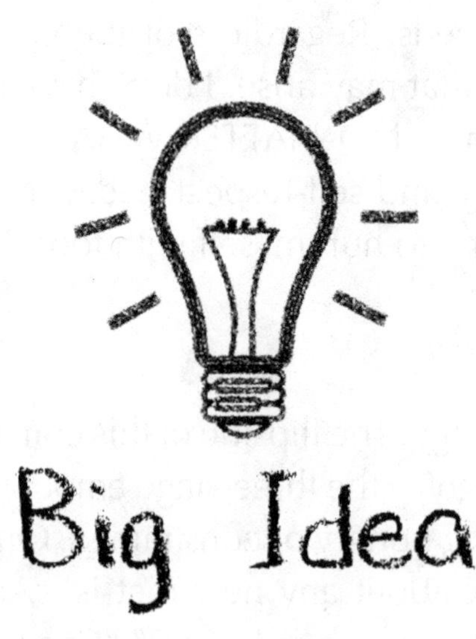

Boundaries don't suppress success, they strengthen and sustain it.

Therefore, the first step in the A,B,C's of "enough" is to *"A"* – **A**ccept the fact that we can live with enough. We'll be perfectly fine eating the right amount. Our need for nutrition is clearly quantifiable. Our desire for more is immeasurable. We need to use food to fuel our body, not use our feelings to fuel our fear of not having enough.

This acceptance is not going to instantaneously carve away the cravings or appease our appetite for more. If we're used to ordering the super-sized sirloin, it's probably going to be disorienting to now just "settle" for six ounces. That sensation is not going to go away overnight. But remember, those are just feelings and not facts. Our head and our heart might not always be aligned, but at least we'll know which should be on top.

The bedrock of our Soveya Solution is to be fueled by facts and not paralyzed by false perceptions. It may very well be uncomfortable in the beginning to "limit" ourselves to the appropriate amounts of food we need instead of feeding our immediate desires – even though the satiation and satisfaction will kick in just a handful of minutes later – as long as we don't grab a few "handfuls" in the meantime.

We're not used to waiting those few uncomfortable moments, but why are we willing to do it anyway? Why are we volunteering to place ourselves in this "predicament"? Because we're buoyed by the first half of "enough is finally enough," which fuels our fortitude to no longer long for the softer, easier way but rather solidifies our courage to do ***whatever it takes*** irrespective of how intimidating or upsetting it appears. Breaking habits simultaneously means breaking old boundaries and building new ones. We're breaking the old boundaries of the fear of deprivation and building new ones based on our objective needs.

And that's how the seeds of true transformation take

root – doing the right thing even though we don't feel like it. We've just taken another step outside our comfort zone into the brave new world of health and wellbeing – and personal growth.

Which brings us to the *"B"* in our A,B,C's of "enough" – ***B***enefit. After a short while, we start to appreciate the benefits of living within boundaries in our relationship with food. We notice the signs of conscientious and consistent weight loss -- how our clothes are not quite as tight and our face not quite as full, and we value waking up in the morning without experiencing the regret and remorse in our heart and the bloated distension in our abdomen. We may still yearn for more sometimes during meals and miss gorging on a huge steak falling off either end of the plate, but we're not fighting it quite as much and we're emotionally more at peace. The food fog is fading and the mental obsession diminishing. We realize that limits are not necessarily limiting but enable us to keep heading in the same direction instead of swerving all over the road and inevitably ending up in the ditch of another binge.

We're improving our health by lowering our blood sugar, A1C, LDL, and HBP (the alphabet soup of suffering) as well continuing to lower the number on the scale. The benefits column on our Clarity List buds like a beautiful spring orchard, serving up the delicious physical and emotional fruits of our progress. We feel much more energetic and we sleep better at night.

Our back doesn't hurt quite as much and we're not out

of breath going up a flight of stairs. Family and friends share compliments and encouragement, and we bask in the inner joy of integrity and self-respect. Is the most delectable double-fudge brownie really worth jeopardizing these gifts and gains? Really? Really?!

And then, sometime in the near or not-so-distant future, we begin **C**elebrating enough – which is the "C" in the A,B,C's of "enough." We can sincerely **c**elebrate enough and engender an earnest emotional joy around the boundaries of our food plan. We can come to the point of actually being repulsed by overeating and no longer value the quality of the meal based solely on the quantity we consume.

We're no longer attracted to that stuffed feeling in our stomach, nor associate comfort or happiness with eating without control. We are free from the compulsion to overeat and have developed healthier coping mechanisms with the challenges that life will inevitably serve up. Or at least, we are no longer comfortable using food as an escape.

Digesting the fundamental principles that inform, enrich, and effectuate the Soveya Solution become part of our regular routine. We're chipping away at the outer crust of apprehension and uncertainty that have covered us for so long and confidently wear the cloak of credibility that fits us so nicely. We're content and committed to do the right thing for us no matter what environment in which we find ourselves – or what other people are doing around us.

Have we become perfect people? Hardly. Our self-growth is about progress, not perfection. But, at the same time, we're poised and prepared to precisely manage our food plan regardless of the internal speed bumps or external detours we may encounter. Our destination is always attainable regardless of the weather or operating conditions.

Our self-care through proper nutrition no matter what the circumstances is just what we do. Because it's a primary priority, that makes it not such a big deal. That's the irony of it all. The more we accept the boundaries, the less we fight. The more we surrender our self-will, the more willingness we gain. The more we engage in the transformation, the less effort we need to expend.

Oh, and by the way, we'll be maintaining a healthy weight as well. Pretty cool!

How long does it take to get to the *C* of the A, B, C's? Well, how long does it take to get to the Tootsie Roll center of a Tootsie Pop? Everyone has their own stopwatch. But these are measurable markers and tangible goals for anyone to attain – and even more importantly, to maintain. And they last a lot longer than those three licks.

The more material these measures mean to us, the more we'll expend effort on a daily basis to ensure they become and remain part and parcel of our personality.

And then it becomes apparent to us that along with having transformed our body size, we have actually transformed the burden of saying "no" into the freedom to say "no." All it took was mastering these simple A,B,C's – which is the culmination of the Seven Soveya Keys.

We are a new person in a new body – and no lobotomy or stomach surgery was necessary. Just the willingness to be unconditionally honest with ourselves and focus on changing our relationship with food instead of just trying to lessen our body size. And the best part of all is that it's a foolproof formula if we don't act foolishly enough to forgo it. It's a rinse and repeat cycle for whatever environment in which we find ourselves, and in whichever stage of life we currently reside.

One day at a time – no matter what, no matter when, no matter where, no matter why and no matter with whom. Because we love and value ourselves and solemnly affirm to preserve and protect our nutritional needs no matter what the circumstances. And at the conclusion of another successful day, we savior the sweetest and most nourishing notion that NOTHING TASTES AS GOOD AS FEELING GOOD FEELS!

"I continue to be very grateful to you, as I truly feel your support and your teachings helped me create a much, much healthier relationship not only with food but with life itself. I also started running again, training for a half marathon. In general, my heart feels very happy. I find myself smiling during the day for no reason or all reasons. I really can't express enough thanks to you."

– Karen, Philadelphia, Pennsylvania

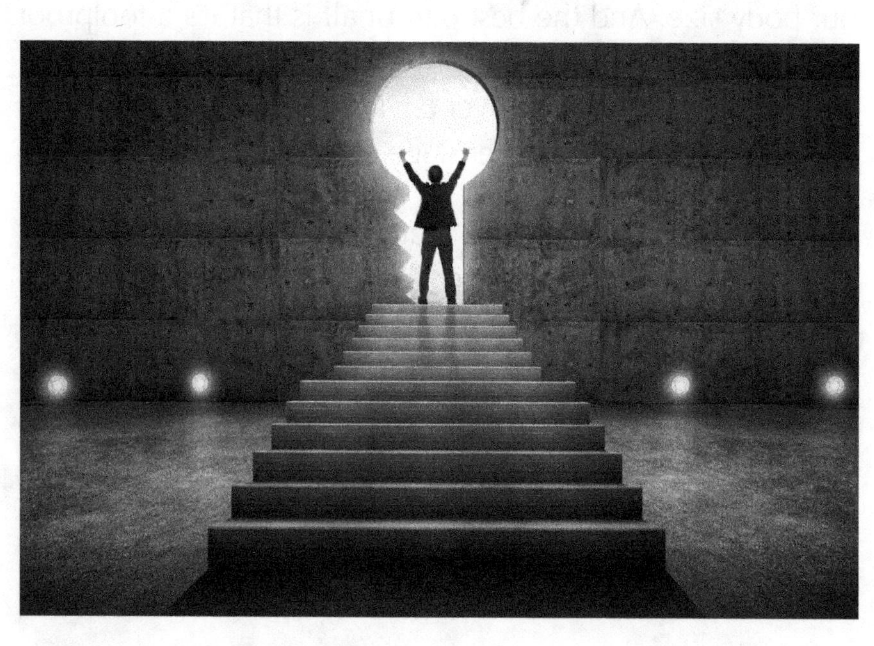

INDEX OF IDEAS

For the sake of helpful review and easy access, here is a list of the primary points and fundamental principles that dot the i's of the Soveya Solution and allow our eyes to keep seeing clearly as we continue on our journey toward developing and maintaining a healthy relationship with food:

THE SOVEYA SOLUTION

- Successful weight loss is not about *losing weight*. It's about developing a *healthy relationship with food*.
- A healthy relationship with food is using food to fuel your body, not feed your feelings.
- It's not about changing your body size – it's about changing yourself.
- Head, heart, and hands are the three target areas of change.
- Eat to live, don't live to eat.
- Obesity is not a *medical* problem – it's a *behavior* problem. It's a temptation, not a tumor.

- It's not a *weight* problem, it's a *food* problem. Focus on the problem, not the consequence.
- Unconditional honesty and self-maturation are the lynchpins for change.

ELI'S STORY

- I was a compulsive overeater. I was utterly overwhelmed by my desire to indulge with food.
- The distance between my head and heart seemed like 18 miles instead of 18 inches. When it came to food, "no" was not in my vocabulary.
- I couldn't differentiate between five ounces and five pounds. I was quantitatively challenged. Enough was never, ever enough.
- I'd use food to reward myself and to distract me from things I didn't want to think about – the perfect anesthetic. Fritos instead of feelings.
- I was more diligent with pizza than pushups. I fiddled with fad diets, endured half-day fasts and dabbled with diet pills. The stimulants didn't magically make me lose weight, just eat faster.
- Maybe I was destined to be fat. Why bother fighting it anymore? Maybe lots and lots was my lot in life.
- The clarity and conviction I had in other aspects of my life completely escaped me when it came to food. Discipline and determination disappeared down a donut hole.
- Completely desperate and humiliated, I finally

acknowledged that I had to stop working on dieting and start working on changing myself.

- I was grasping at external solutions for an internal problem. That's why I could never get a grip.
- I had a palpable fear of feeling restricted and deprived. I was enslaved by my entitlement to indulge.
- I accepted the challenge of unconditional honesty. I felt at ease and emotionally prepared to do whatever it took to CHANGE my relationship with food, not just to try and lose weight. I was ready to say "no." Enough was finally enough.

THE FOOD PLAN

- If you fail to plan, then you're planning to fail.
- Inspiration doesn't change us, it just shows direction. We have to take the steps.
- Intuitive eating doesn't work. Our intuition is broken when it comes to food. It's not an asset, it's a liability.
- Our vision is always askew when it comes to food.
- The food plan is the corrective lenses that allows us to successfully travel toward our weight-loss destination, avoiding the hazards and pitfalls that have littered our path up to this point.
- Feelings are not facts. Act on hunger, not appetite.
- Hunger is our body's need for proper nutrition. Appetite is our spontaneous desire to use food for physical enjoyment, indulgence, comfort, or any

other perceived momentary benefit, the most common being stress relief or emotional eating.

- The function of food is fuel for our body. Quality, quantity, and timing are the three criteria for healthy fueling.
- Focus on nutrients, not calories: protein, carbohydrates, lipids (fats), vitamins, minerals, water.
- Function should not *rule out* fun, it should *rule over* fun. The pleasure of eating is a wonderful benefit, but not its underlying purpose.
- I had to stop rationalizing and justifying my immediate desire to indulge, and to be willing to grow up – and grow out of the "six-year-old syndrome" – that just because I felt that I wanted to eat didn't necessarily mean that was the right choice for me to make at that moment.
- The food plan gave me the 20/20 vision to navigate my way through my daily nutrition, helping me differentiate between feelings and facts, between hunger and appetite.
- The stronger the boundaries, the easier the effort and the greater the success.
- Eating to meet our body's needs has measurable limits, but feeding our feelings is often a bottomless pit.
- Whether we're overwhelmed, overworked, stressed, or fatigued, our food plan will be the bedrock of consistency and accountability, where we would otherwise be much more susceptible to spontaneously succumb to sudden temptation.
- Eat to your fill, not till your full.

- Satiation is a learned skill, not necessarily a naturally occurring feeling.
- I had to learn how to nourish myself instead of indulging myself.
- I had to take the pain to the make the gain – or in this case, lose the weight.
- Nothing tastes as good as feeling good feels.

STAY INSIDE THE BLUE BOX

- Compulsive eating is an addiction to both a substance and a process.
- Consuming sugar (and most refined carbs) stimulates the brain's reward system, releasing pleasure sensors such as endorphins and dopamine, creating a compulsive craving for more.
- Good carbs vs. bad carbs and robust calories vs. empty calories.
- The fewer the ingredients and/or the added sweeteners, the better the choice.
- The DNA of a craving is twofold: 1) The emotional currency we invest in that immediate physical gratification and; 2) The perception of the profound deprivation and loss if we don't have it.
- Emotional maturity is the ability to process a feeling, not be overwhelmed and overrun by it.
- We have to be willing to step outside of our comfort zone to try new foods and resensitize our tastes to the naturally occurring flavors that inherently exist in less refined and processed options.

- Proactive abstinence vs. passive abstention.
- Compulsive eating is re-engaged if we reconnect those wires of spontaneity and give ourselves permission to act on a momentary desire, no matter how subtle or serious the digression might seem.
- Precision, not perfection.
- The Three Reinforcements after a successful day: 1) We don't regret it; 2) We physically feel good and feel good about ourselves; 3) It wasn't as hard as we thought.
- The primary purpose of the food plan is to create a method and medium to achieve proactive and long-term abstinence and freedom from compulsive eating.

KEY ONE: C.H.A.N.G.E.

- Nothing changes if nothing changes.
- The opposite of pleasure is comfort, not pain.
- Progress instead of paralysis.
- To the extent of the effort is the reward.
- Change stimulates growth. Complacency cause stagnation.
- C.H.A.N.G.E. stands for: ***C***ourage, ***H***umility, ***A***ccountability, ***N***ecessity, ***G***ratitude, ***E***nthusiasm.
- ***C***ourage is the necessary first step toward change because we need the courage to confront and conquer our comfort zone.
- One small step of progress often requires a giant leap of faith in ourselves.

- We need humility to engender the willingness to be teachable at whatever age, stage, and station of life we're in – to welcome and embrace change and learn new behaviors.
- Engaging unconditional honesty in confronting detrimental attitudes, obsessions, and fixations with food is crucial in allowing the underpinnings of change to take hold. And humility is the foundation upon which honesty can root.
- We'll work harder and push ourselves more if someone is standing over us. Being pulled past our comfort zone is a much smaller step than if we have to leap it on our own – even though it's really the same distance.
- The three A's for effective coaching: Advocacy, Accountability, and Action.
- For years I was the reigning monarch of rationalization when it came to giving in to my obsession with self-indulgence.
- Wisdom means being able to tell the difference between what's important and what's *more* important.
- The most important responsibility we have every day is managing our own health.
- Changing your relationship with food – being willing to do whatever is necessary to heal your body from being overweight or obese and to break lifelong habits – has to be your primary priority, day in and day out.
- Adopting an attitude of gratitude and lighting a fire of enthusiasm are essential for sustained success.

- We resent having to change – having to put limits on ourselves. We're bitter about having to eat vegetables, even if they aren't bitter herbs.
- Be comfortable being temporarily uncomfortable.
- Feel the freedom to say "no" instead of feeling burdened to say "no."
- Enthusiastically embrace the effort, don't be burdened by the bitterness.
- "Whatever it takes!"

KEY TWO: H.A.L.T.

- Just because we're hungry doesn't mean we need to eat.
- Hydrate and contemplate – drink and think, don't feel and flail.
- H.A.L.T. stands for: ***H***ungry, ***A***ngry, ***L***onely, ***T***ired. These are the four universal situations in life that either create a craving and/or which we associate with eating.
- A "healthy" feeling of hunger is when the glucose levels in our cells begin to diminish, resulting in a lack of energy which stimulates a sensation in the body to refuel. It's a legitimate need for nutrition.
- Vulnerability doesn't have to equate inevitability – just because we're compromised doesn't mean we have to cave in.
- The car is not going to stop on its own. But just because I'm hungry, that doesn't mean I need to lay the pedal to the metal. And upon giving myself those

few minutes to digest the food and "step away from the plate," the sensation of satiation will start slowing down the momentum and take the edge off my drive for more.

- The focus of this key is to build the skills of intellectual anticipation and behavioral response to an impending susceptibility, so our actions don't have to replay the same regretful reaction.
- Anger or anxiety, stress or sadness, disappointment or displeasure – these are common expressions of emotional discomfort and turmoil.
- Food is fuel, not a friend. It's not a therapist and it's not a Band-Aid.
- Downtime meant dinner time – even if I had already packed away a full supper.
- We can learn to enjoy our own company, and better enjoy the company of others, if we're not confounded and consumed by thoughts of consuming.
- That's the senseless, self-destructive pattern: we isolate because of our perceived inferiority fueled largely by our large size, which creates a lack of friendship or comfort to commingle with others, which triggers a sensation for food to fill the void of loneliness.
- If I was tired, I needed rest, not raisin bran.
- Following a well-regimented food plan, day after day, helped me rework the wires in my brain that boundaries weren't binding, but building – even if it went against my immediate inclinations.

KEY THREE: F.E.A.R.

- ***F***alse ***E***vidence ***A***ppearing ***R***eal
- Fear-based inaction is one of the primary spike strips that flatten our tires and incapacitate us from making real progress down the road of recovery.
- Throwing away that security blanket of spontaneity that has "shielded" us for so long is demonstrably disconcerting.
- Whether eating is our pacifier, protector, or primary port of unbridled pleasure, ridding ourselves of these behaviors is a Himalayan climb which we feel woefully inadequate to crest.
- Spontaneity is not a sanctuary. Impulsivity doesn't provide immunity to life's challenges. Unrestrained quantities don't result in uninhibited pleasure, just a momentary thrill followed by extended anguish.
- We're paralyzed by our perceptions instead of fueled by facts.
- Evidence rooted in subjective perceptions that appears real to us isn't always so. In fact, it's often false. Learning to walk through – and work through -- our fears is an emboldening and elevating experience – even with the requisite discomfort.
- The first flicker of hunger triggers an alarm, creating a convoluted conclusion that we can't withstand the next few minutes without satisfying that sensation.
- Hydrate and contemplate. Drink and think; don't feel and flail.
- Drink some water and process the feeling. Wait

those five uncomfortable minutes for the sensation to simmer down and the water to saturate inside. Work it through, don't let it work you over.

- By feeding our irrationality, we continue to sanction spontaneity under the guise of a necessary reaction to a temporary discomfort, which perpetuates the problem instead of seeding the solution.
- Only by putting blinders on our skewed vision will we be able to move forward and walk through our fears. In our mind's eye it seems like the edge of a cliff, when in actuality it's the first few steps toward real freedom.

KEY FOUR: FACE YOUR STUFF, DON'T STUFF YOUR FACE

- The pebble is a pain, but it's not incapacitating. A man with a pebble in his shoe will deal with it until he can deal with it – he's not going to debilitate himself to deal with a discomfort, nor anesthetize himself to alleviate an annoyance.
- Fritos instead of feelings.
- Food is probably the most universally accessed anesthetic. We eat to sedate our stress, distract our discomfort, placate our pain, and even numb our everyday nuisances.
- We use food as a sweet and soothing sedative. It's not *like* a drug. It *IS* a drug – the most abused drug in the world. It's legal, easily available, and more

proactively promoted than any other licit or illicit contraband around.

- We're rash to rationalize our self-diagnoses, secure in the fact that we can always write our own prescription.
- Eating over a problem leaves us with two problems.
- The prize in the Cracker-Jack box doesn't contain the solution for our difficulties. There are no answers in the Almond Joy, and polishing off a pint of Rocky Road doesn't ease our path – remaining true to its name.
- The act of self-medicating to sedate stress is destructive and debilitating, further seeding the sequence of escape and avoidance of seeking solutions.
- Our goal is not to feel good for the moment – no matter the consequence – but to release our stress in a productive manner that leaves us better off at the end, not worse off.
- Having someone to talk to, or a physical activity in which to engage, doesn't necessarily resolve the core issue. But it serves the incredibly constructive function of exorcising that negative emotional energy. Sports, walking, running, yoga, meditating, talking, and journaling are just some examples of highly useful and easily accessible vehicles of release.
- Stuffing down our feelings with an apple strudel just adds to the angst as soon as the serotonin from the sugar subsides, leaving us with a hardened heart and bloated belly.
- Purge, don't plunge. We need to purge our stress, not plunge it down with food.

- Competitive eating is a growing sport at the same time as weight gain and obesity are among the primary sources accounting for the skyrocketing cost of health care. Diabetes has been designated as the fastest-growing disease in the history of modern medicine.
- Abstinence has to be intrinsic, not dependent.
- "This too shall pass." Stay on the bus, because the scenery will change. Our feelings are also fluid.
- It's okay to feel our feelings. It's never okay to feed them.
- We can all muster the courage to face our stuff and not stuff our face if we maintain the clarity of consequence and the belief in the benefit.
- We can realize that the power inside of us is always stronger than the problem in front of us. And if we are of a spiritual nature, then the Power above us is certainly greater than the problem in front of us.
- Power down your projected expectations on others and unleash the incredible power you have inside yourself to meet your remarkable potential.
- Surrender equals serenity. Surrender doesn't mean giving in, and it certainly doesn't mean giving up. It means giving it over. We need to give up emotional control of those things – and people – over which we have no control.
- The more we accept the things we cannot change (others) and focusing on changing the things we can (ourselves) the more emotional serenity we'll develop, and the less disposed we'll be toward emotional eating.

KEY FIVE: TODAY IS THE CURE FOR THE DIS-EASE OF TOMORROW

- The "disease" of tomorrow is a promising pillow of procrastination on which to rest our raging rationalizations, giving us solace to succumb to our immediate inclinations – even though it will end up being nothing more than an agonizing bed of nails.
- It's dis-eased thinking – a dearth of direct and deliberate discernment when confronted with a desire for a Danish.
- We invest our emotional energy into the fear of the future which paralyzes us from being successful in the present.
- The disease of tomorrow is the perception that ***today*** we need to possess the strength and acuity to bear the burden of successfully fulfilling our future accomplishments.
- Our head may strategize over a twelve-month span, but we need to keep the schedule in our heart locked on the daily view.
- Stay in the day!
- Every morning our reservoir is restocked with a sufficient supply of emotional currency to spend for that next day. That's one of the incredible functions of sleep. It allows us to reframe, refocus, re-energize and recharge. It's a daily direct deposit in our determination account.
- We have no time machine nor predictive powers

to accurately ascertain the degree of our future fortitude and mental makeup. So, why in the world would we allow a mindset about which we have no clue inform and guide our attitude today?

- Taking it one day at a time is the only express train with the best chance of getting you to your destination on time.
- If tomorrow you employ the same tools and take the same actions that produced a healthy and productive relationship with food today, there's a darn good chance you'll get the same results.
- Long-term success is nothing more than an accumulation of daily accomplishments.
- So many times, our momentary subjective fears massage a manageable molehill into a massive mountainside, convincing us that we have no choice but to detour directly to the donuts.
- The *perception* of the degree of difficulty is 99% of the time greater than the *actual* degree of difficulty. It's not as hard as we think.
- The more often we apply the key of TODAY in our daily eating encounters, we'll tellingly transform our entire outlook and relationship with food.
- If it ain't broke, don't fix it.
- During the past seventeen years, I can say with unwavering clarity that I have never regretted any choices I made that continued to build and bolster my abstinence.
- If we plan to take care of our food plan, the food plan will take care of us.
- If we stay in the day, the abstinence will stay in us.

KEY SIX: CLARITY IS KEY

- When we enter any challenging food environment, our success is severely handicapped if we don't have a firm hold on our clarity.
- It's our pocket umbrella that keeps us from getting wet in a sudden storm. Because, when it comes to our propensity to pardon a piece of pecan pie, there's always a forecast for rain in our brain.
- The forethought is the mental gymnastics we so eloquently execute to excuse the éclair.
- No sooner do we polish off the last bite then we are pained with the somber reality that "I didn't need to eat that. I can't believe I did it again."
- The afterthought is the objective reality, while the forethought is the subjective justification.
- Our goal is to maintain the clarity of the afterthought ***at the time*** of the forethought.
- The Clarity List. Consequences and Benefits. By creating a chart and populating these two columns, we give ourselves the ability to see clearly and stay in our lane when the rain begins to fog our windshield and reduce our visibility.
- Whereas when it was on our plate, our vision was locked in to the confines of the four square inches of fudge-covered cake, we now can see beyond the last bite, and all the crumbs of crummy consequences that predictably trail behind.
- We have to capture that clarity and house it in our hand-held flashlight, which we need to manually

turn on and illuminate our path each day. Because when it comes to our relationship with food, our honesty power plant often suffers random blackouts.

- Utilizing the Clarity List in the context of a flu shot is much more effective and impactful than merely trying to rely on it as an antibiotic.
- Once we are triggered with a craving, it's much harder to first start building up our emotional immune system on the spot when already confronted with the cheesecake. It's like trying to affix the storm shutters to our windows when the winds have already reached gale-force strength. It's usually a losing battle.
- We need to take our flu shots *before* we're compromised. We need to put up the shutters while it's still sunny. The calm before the storm is when the successful preparations take place.
- We're learning to live life between meals without food - without the ever-present possibility of grazing, noshing, bingeing, or grabbing.
- The Clarity List continually creates a fresh platform of honesty and objectivity upon which to accurately assess the cost of deviating from our food plan.
- It's not about the momentary caloric intake or lack of nutritional value. It has nothing to do with counting points or calculating ketosis. It's all about changing our behavior. And succumbing to this "one-time" impulse just continues to pump the heartbeat of our compulsion.
- Our bright and bold boundaries are on the forefront

of our mind, allowing us to maintain the clarity of the afterthought at the time of the forethought. We're securely tethered to the truth while tempted with the tiramisu.

- The flu shot doesn't dissipate the virus, it just guards us from being infected. The umbrella doesn't clear away the clouds, it just protects us from getting wet. So too, the Clarity List doesn't disintegrate the donuts, it just helps us dispel the notion that it's too hard, too uncomfortable, too tempting, or too depriving to do without.
- Our vulnerability no longer has to equate inevitability.

KEY SEVEN: ENOUGH IS ENOUGH

- Transform the burden of saying "no" into the freedom to say "no."
- Are you sick and tired of being sick and tired?
- The difference between being 99% willing and 100% willing is not 1%, it's 1,000%.
- Some people change when they see the light. Most people change when they feel the heat.
- What are you going to do today? Whatever it takes!
- You are worth investing in your health and wellbeing. You are worth prioritizing your needs.
- No matter what, you're not going to overeat today.
- We have a palpable fear of feeling restricted. We feel so boxed-in by boundaries that we're ready to burst.

- Putting limits on our eating habits is not a necessary evil – but necessarily enabling. Boundaries don't suppress success they strengthen and sustain it.
- A, B, C's of "enough: ***A***ccept, ***B***enefit, **C**elebrate.
- Our need for nutrition is clearly quantifiable. Our desire for more is immeasurable.
- The bedrock of the Soveya Solution is to be fueled by facts and not paralyzed by false perceptions.
- Breaking habits simultaneously means breaking old boundaries and building new ones.
- We notice the signs of conscientious and consistent weight loss -- how our clothes are not quite as tight and our face not quite as full, and we value waking up in the morning without experiencing the regret and remorse in our heart and the bloated distension in our abdomen.
- The food fog is fading and the mental obsession diminishing.
- The benefits column on our Clarity List buds like a beautiful spring orchard, serving up the delicious physical and emotional fruits of our progress.
- We can actually **c**elebrate enough and engender an earnest emotional joy around the boundaries of our food plan and no longer value the quality of the meal based solely on the quantity we consume.
- We're content and committed to do the right thing for us no matter what environment in which we find ourselves – or what other people are doing around us.
- The more we accept the boundaries, the less we

fight. The more we surrender our self-will, the more willingness we gain. The more we engage in the transformation, the less effort we need to expend.

- The more material these measures mean to us, the more we'll expend effort on a daily basis to ensure they become and remain part and parcel of our personality.
- Besides from having transformed our body size, we have actually transformed the burden of saying "no" into the freedom to say "no."
- One day at a time – no matter what, no matter when, no matter where, no matter why, and no matter with whom.
- Because NOTHING TASTES AS GOOD AS FEELING GOOD FEELS!

"Thank you for helping me the past twenty weeks I've worked with you. You have helped me overcome so many obstacles that I wouldn't have been able to overcome myself. It was a pleasure working with you, and I'm so happy that I did."

- N.D., Las Vegas, Nevada

fight. The more we surrender our self-will, the more willingness we gain. The more we engage in the transformation, the less effort we need to expend.

- The more material these measures mean to us, the more we'll expend effort on a daily basis to ensure they become and remain part and parcel of our personality.
- Besides from having transformed our body size, we have actually transformed the burden of saying "no" into the freedom to say "no."
- One day at a time – no matter what, no matter when, no matter where, no matter why, and no matter with whom.
- Because NOTHING TASTES AS GOOD AS FEELING GOOD FEELS!

"Thank you for helping me the past twenty weeks I've worked with you. You have helped me overcome so many obstacles that I wouldn't have been able to overcome myself. It was a pleasure working with you, and I'm so happy that I did."

- N.D., Las Vegas, Nevada

- Putting limits on our eating habits is not a necessary evil – but necessarily enabling. Boundaries don't suppress success they strengthen and sustain it.
- A, B, C's of "enough: ***A***ccept, ***B***enefit, **C**elebrate.
- Our need for nutrition is clearly quantifiable. Our desire for more is immeasurable.
- The bedrock of the Soveya Solution is to be fueled by facts and not paralyzed by false perceptions.
- Breaking habits simultaneously means breaking old boundaries and building new ones.
- We notice the signs of conscientious and consistent weight loss -- how our clothes are not quite as tight and our face not quite as full, and we value waking up in the morning without experiencing the regret and remorse in our heart and the bloated distension in our abdomen.
- The food fog is fading and the mental obsession diminishing.
- The benefits column on our Clarity List buds like a beautiful spring orchard, serving up the delicious physical and emotional fruits of our progress.
- We can actually **c**elebrate enough and engender an earnest emotional joy around the boundaries of our food plan and no longer value the quality of the meal based solely on the quantity we consume.
- We're content and committed to do the right thing for us no matter what environment in which we find ourselves – or what other people are doing around us.
- The more we accept the boundaries, the less we

EATING TO SATISFACTION IS THE GREATEST BLESSING

soveya

so·*VEY*·ah

Soveya is a Hebrew word meaning **satisfied**. It's often found in the Torah (the Jewish Bible) as well as Talmudic teachings in the context of eating.

One of the primary sources is in the book of Deuteronomy (*Devarim*), chapter 8, verse 10: *"And you will eat, and you will be satisfied, and you will bless the Lord."*

The fundamental values we derive from this verse can inform and enrich our relationship with food. And as you'll see, this is why I chose the name Soveya.

I'll focus on three words in the sentence: to *eat*; to be *satisfied*; and to *bless*.

To ***eat***. The purpose of eating is to provide our bodies with the essential nutrients we need to survive. Take away our food, and we will die. It's that simple. Therefore, eating -- by definition -- should be an act that brings health, vitality, and life to a person.

If we engage in acts of eating that run contrary to that goal, we are causing ourselves harm instead of health and are not fulfilling the function of food for which it was intended. As the classic scholar Maimonides wrote more than 1,000 years ago: "Overeating is like poison for anyone and it is the primary cause of all illness. Most illnesses are caused either by eating harmful foods or overeating even healthy foods." (*Laws of Knowledge*, Chapter 4, paragraph 15).

To be ***satisfied***: We are directed to eat in order to satisfy our body's need for nutrition and sustenance, to provide us the energy and well-being to carry out our purpose in this world. As we have all experienced, eating beyond this point is an easy and alluring trap into which to fall. Food is tempting and tastes good; it provides comfort, convenience, and an emotional elixir for stress and anxiety. It might make us momentarily merry, but we're left much less than satisfied.

To ***bless***: If we're able to maintain our boundaries, make the right choices, and eat the right amounts, we're left feeling extremely grateful, content, and satisfied. The fact that the food was flavorsome, appetizing, and a physically enjoyable experience adds greatly to our gratification.

We're commanded to capture that moment and use it as a springboard for appreciation – to recognize that food is an incredibly special and vital gift for us to preserve our health and to acknowledge the Source from where it originated.

Connecting these three ideas certainly helps concretize the concept that eating to satisfaction is truly one of the greatest blessings.

"It has been a year and a half since I started working with Soveya, and you have completely changed my life. I lost about twenty-five pounds over the first few months and was able to maintain it. Six weeks ago, I had a baby. I only gained eighteen pounds during the pregnancy and lost it within a few weeks of my baby's birth. She is now six weeks old, and I am profoundly grateful for all the work you do since I was able to wear all my regular clothing almost right away. Whenever people comment I always tell them about you."

- Deborah, Brooklyn, New York

CPSIA information can be obtained
at www.ICGtesting.com
Printed in the USA
BVHW040654240520
580221BV00008B/152

9 781478 764885